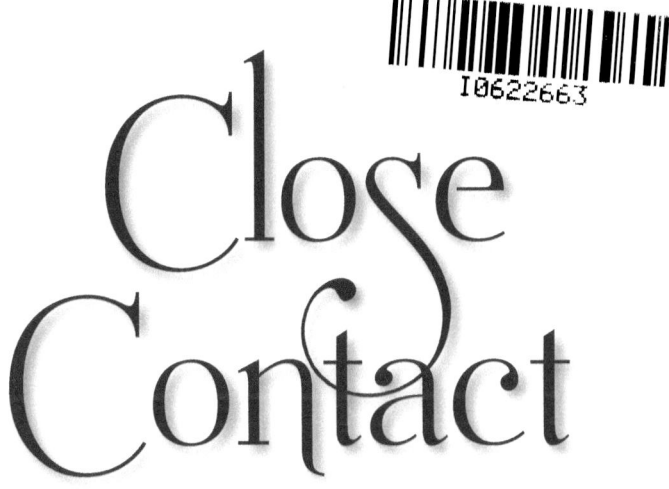

Close Contact

*Memoir of a
Determined Pandemic
Cancer Survivor*

WENDY ORMSBY

3 Cs
Press

Published by 3 Cs Press

Produced by GMK Writing and Editing, Inc.
Managing Editor: Katie Benoit
Edited by Laura Oliver
Proofread by Kelly Clody
Text design and composition by Libby Kingsbury
Cover design by Libby Kingsbury
Cover photo, *Chincoteague Sunset,* by Wendy Ormsby
Printed by IngramSpark

Print ISBN: 979-8-9883417-3-4
Ebook EISN: 979-8-9883417-4-1

Visit the author at:
  www.wendyormsby.com
  www.ormsbygraphics.com
  linkedin.com/in/wendyormsby/

Note: This publication is presented solely for informational, educational, and entertainment purposes. It is not intended to provide personal, health, relationship, legal, financial, or other advice and should not be relied upon as such. If expert assistance is required, the services of a professional should be sought.

Success is liking yourself, liking what you do,
and liking how you do it.

—Maya Angelou

To my dear friend, Colleen Heitkamp, for unknowingly putting my cancer into perspective while sharing her own personal life challenges.

Acknowledgments

I would like to start by thanking my husband, Mark Ormsby. He has always been there for me physically, mentally, emotionally, and spiritually, especially during my active cancer treatments. I could not have done it without him. In addition, I would like to thank my forever friend, Julie Deller. She always knows just what to say to pick me up when I'm feeling down.

Along with them, I would like to thank my friend, Jonathan Freeman-Coppadge, for his great writing class and for introducing me to my amazing editor, Laura Oliver. Her many encouraging words and much appreciated honesty made my story come to life in the best way possible. And thank you to Alesha Peluso, my marketing and platform coach, who helped me get my story out there.

Contents

Author's Note

I decided to write my story about having breast cancer during the coronavirus (COVID-19) pandemic early on in my treatments. I was having trouble working with a doctor and was hoping that, if I took notes on our visits, things would make more sense to me.

As time passed, I experienced so many struggles with the treatments that I became determined to write down my thoughts, so I could share my situation with others who have had similar struggles or know someone else who has.

I sincerely hope you will benefit from reading my story, as a patient or a loved one, no matter where you are in your cancer endeavor.

I wish you, your family, your friends, and the rest of your community the best of health and happiness. May we never have to deal with the trials and tribulations of a pandemic again.

That Call

IT'S EARLY EVENING ON JANUARY 8, 2020. I KNOW IT CAN TAKE UP to six days to get the biopsy results. I have already been waiting six full days to hear from Dr. B.

As the six o'clock hour on the sixth day approaches, I become more convinced that I will have to wait yet another day. Of course, this means another sleepless night ahead of me.

My husband, Mark, is not home from work yet. Our oldest and youngest are getting their showers, and our middle child is engrossed in her homework at the dining room table. I'm doing my best to distract myself as I read the same line over and over in my book. I should be starting dinner, but my focus on that call prevents even a hint of that from happening.

The phone rings, and I recognize my doctor's name on the caller ID. Dr. B had done my annual breast exams for the past twelve years. I'm both afraid of what she will say and relieved that I no longer need to prolong the agony. Although I have been keeping the phone nearby long before 6 p.m., I wait for a couple of rings before I answer it.

"H…Hello?"

"Hi, is this Wendy Ormsby?" Dr. B asks.

"Yes, it is." My voice is unsteady.

"I have your biopsy results from last week," she continues. "You have invasive mammary carcinoma."

What language is she speaking?

I strain to decipher each word. I know "mammary" is the body part affected. And "carcinoma" sounds like cancer. However, the word "invasive" is buzzing around in my head like a mosquito drawn to a bug zapper.

My response to Dr. B is not at all what I was expecting.

No matter how prepared I thought I might be, that no longer matters.

I'm frozen.

I swear I'm uttering something in response. Then I realize I'm not saying a word.

"You have breast cancer," she confirms.

I feel my heart throbbing in my chest. Words are still escaping me.

As she continues talking, it's as if I am watching the whole scenario from across the room. The word "cancer" fills my mind, leaving room for nothing else.

"Is there anyone else in the room with you?" she asks.

No matter how hard I try, I still can't speak. If I can just get a quick drink of water then, maybe, I can talk. I only need a minute.

She waits in silence.

Finally, I take a deep breath. "My daughter…Erin is here."

"Hand the phone to Erin."

Wait. What?

Erin is sometimes mature beyond her years, but this is too much for a high school sophomore to absorb.

Still struggling to speak, I hand the phone to Erin anyway then step into the kitchen for some water. As I'm taking small sips, and trying to breathe normally again, I overhear Dr. B on the phone with Erin.

"She'll need a bilateral MRI," she says.

I quickly take the phone from Erin and let Dr. B know that I am back and ready to talk. If she is planning on telling Erin the next steps, then I need to continue the call with her myself.

Deep down inside, I feel that what my children know about my cancer should ultimately be up to me. Of course, I won't keep vital information from them. Still, my innate mothering sense tells me to protect my children. If there is anything they do not need to know, then why worry them even more?

As Dr. B is telling me what will happen next, I grab a pen and anxiously scribble some notes in a nearby notebook. Otherwise, I know there is no way I'll remember anything.

I hang up the phone, and Mark walks in the front door.

I'm calm but choking back tears.

He sees me sitting on the couch with my hands on my face and my head down. A similar look to when my grandmother passed away. I look up at him and see in his eyes he already knows. I stand up and we hug.

My oldest child comes up from the basement and notices

I'm upset. Erin enters the room and, even though she didn't quite follow what my doctor said on the phone, her teared-up eyes tell me she already knows.

"I have cancer," I say, trying to keep my composure.

My oldest gives me a firm but gentle hug as if saying everything will be okay. I'm thinking that this is no way for a senior to spend the last semester of high school.

Despite my cancer diagnosis, I can't help but notice how strong and brave the four of us are at this moment, considering none of us know what the near future holds. Maybe it isn't quite sinking in yet. However, it's obvious we are all in this together.

* * *

Before my MRI appointment day arrives, I decide to start researching breast cancer treatment options. I feel overwhelmed with mixed emotions as I type in the words "breast cancer treatments" on my computer. I can't believe this pertains to me personally. Still, I want to know everything I can about it so I will be mentally prepared for anything.

Turns out it isn't such a good idea after all. Reading as much as possible on this subject can be quite daunting. Plus, there is so much more to it than just a breast cancer diagnosis. It might be best to wait until I meet with my oncologist.

While I'm still on the internet, I come across a subject that keeps grabbing the headlines. It's the virus that was first detected in Wuhan, China. This virus is compared to the SARS outbreak in 2003. I remember reading about SARS—severe acute respiratory syndrome—back then and thinking how lucky many of us were at the time. How fewer than fifty cases were found in the United States and none of those patients died.

For some reason, the thought of this new virus makes me nervous, though. Perhaps because, this time, I'm facing uncertain cancer challenges. I'm hoping this virus gets under control at least as quickly as the one in 2003.

- 2 -

Appetite and Insight

EARLY NOVEMBER 2019 WAS WHEN I FIRST NOTICED SOMETHING unusual. It was only eight months after receiving my annual mammogram results saying, "No mammographic evidence of malignancy." It didn't matter what the results said. I knew something had changed since then. The question is, was it anything to worry about?

I wasn't looking for anything unusual. However, something did stand out to me. It also seemed like it wasn't there the day before. At that time, my daily morning routine consisted of a shower, breakfast, then helping my husband make sure everyone was off to school on time.

As I was lathering up in the shower, I felt an unusual shape on my left breast. Over the years, I've heard women say, "I found a lump." Of course, that's not something I had ever expected in my life personally. Probably nobody does. Well, the unusual shape was what I'd call a lump.

Next, I checked the right side to see if it felt the same.

Nope. Then, I went back to the left side to see if maybe I was mistaken the first time.

It was no mistake.

I had already been performing monthly breast checks for many years and never found anything suspicious until that day. I had also been losing weight since the previous year due to having trouble eating with a painful tooth. Maybe it had become clearer once I lost weight.

To this day, I'm not sure why I waited a few weeks to do anything about it. Perhaps it was denial on my part. Or maybe I was just making sure that there was really something wrong.

Either way, with major holidays approaching, the thought of having cancer was weighing heavily on my mind. About a week before Thanksgiving, I talked to Mark about it.

"I think I found a lump," I said. My hands started shaking. I had to sit down. "I'm not even sure there's anything wrong," I continued. "Would you mind checking too? If you find it easily, then I'll know it isn't just my imagination."

Talk about denial.

Sure enough, he found it too. As scary as it was, it was time to make an appointment.

As I was dialing the number for Dr. B's office, I started thinking about how I was going to make that appointment. What exactly do I tell them? How do I describe what's going on with me? It rang a few times, then I heard a woman's voice on the other end.

"How can I help you?" she asked.

"Uh, hi. I need to make an appointment with my doctor."

"What seems to be the problem?"

"I, uh… I found a lump." My stomach fluttered.

"Where did you find it?"

"Um… It's on my breast."

"Which side is it on?"

"It's… on the left side." My stomach went from flutters to knots.

As I thought about it, I realized that considering that was nothing new at that office, and the awkwardness was brief, it was worth it. I finished filling her in and then made the appointment. The soonest I could see Dr. B was mid-December.

* * *

Waiting for my appointment day made it especially difficult to enjoy Thanksgiving, my favorite holiday of the year. Mark and I have always prepared holiday meals together. Since I had a lot on my mind this time around, he was an even bigger help with our special dinner.

My family also attended our annual get-together with longtime friends we have considered family and even refer to as "framily." My good friend Trica hosts these gatherings in her home. Although I certainly have no regrets about continuing our traditions, both celebrations were challenging considering my circumstances.

* * *

My appointment day with Dr. B finally arrived. As I was lying there with a paper gown from the waist up, my mind was racing. Unlike the previous twelve years I had had breast exams, that time I heard my own uneasy breathing, and my heart was pounding like a bass drum. So many questions were forming.

Does the fact that my sister had breast cancer mean that my chance of having it increases? If I do have cancer, then how early are we catching it? Has it spread?

"It feels more like a cyst to me," said Dr. B as she examined me.

Not what I expected her to say. For a few seconds, I was relieved. I hoped that maybe this was nothing after all. Maybe this would be the only appointment I'd need.

"We should get it checked out just in case," she continued. "You should get an ultrasound exam done soon. If something does show up on the image, the sonogram, then you'll need a biopsy to see if it's cancer."

I took some deep breaths.

Before I left her office, Dr. B scheduled an appointment for me with a radiologist a few hours later. Again, not what I had expected. Something told me she had picked up on my anxious energy.

At my radiology appointment, I was again lying there gowned from the waist up. After showing the radiology tech where the lump was, she started my ultrasound exam. The monitor was behind my head, so I stretched my neck and looked up to see what she was observing.

I won't pretend to know how to interpret a sonogram, but what I could see was painfully obvious to me. The tech headed out of the room to get the radiologist. I decided to sit up and look more closely at the monitor. That was not a good idea. As I was trying not to get too anxious about it, the tension grew while I stared at the image on the sonogram.

I could not take my eyes off the image. It looked like a dark oval-shaped spot in my breast, and that spot had measurements attached to it!

The fact that she had something to measure scared me enough, let alone how big that spot looked. The tech and radiologist entered the room and asked me to lie back down so they could check me again. As the tech slowly moved the probe around, the radiologist looked at the monitor.

"Wow! That's big! That's really big!" the radiologist said.

Now, if I had been in his shoes, I would have chosen better words to inform me. As unprofessional as his comments were, at least there was some confirmation about my status.

Once I realized that confirmation, tears slowly started rolling down my face. Instead of comforting me, the radiologist made another poor remark.

"Now, let's not get ahead of ourselves here!"

"How do you expect me to react?" I glared at him. "She thought it was only a cyst. It doesn't sound like that to me."

"Who thought it was only a cyst?" His tone was condescending.

"My doctor from this morning."

"We don't know if it's cancer or not. You'll have to get a biopsy done first."

At that point, I just wanted to get out of there. He told me to make an appointment for a biopsy soon, then we were finally done.

* * *

As Christmas drew closer, I tried more and more to only think about celebrating with family and friends. Up to this point, my husband and I were still the only ones who knew that I could possibly be living with cancer. Along with that, word was getting out about that potentially deadly virus spreading throughout China.

As I ran around trying to get the last of my Christmas shopping done, my mind wandered. What kind of year would 2020 be for me? And for my family? If I did have cancer and ended up feeling incredibly sick from it, who would take care of things around the house?

I had spent the previous forty years of my life taking care of others. I started babysitting the neighborhood kids when I was eleven. I was a professional nanny for twelve years after that. I also worked with children with special needs in school and therapeutic settings for several years and had been a volunteer preschool teacher at Cedar Ridge Community Church where my family attends. Not to mention, Mark and I were raising our own kids.

As for my graphic design business, finding clients when I was healthy was challenging enough, let alone if I had cancer.

Our kids were mostly self-sufficient. Though Mark's job kept him busy, he was always as helpful as he could be. If we asked our older two to help us more around the house or with the dogs, they would.

So, then what was I really worried about?

* * *

We didn't travel anywhere for that Christmas because it would've been too exhausting for five of us to drive over four hundred miles to the closest relatives. Not to mention, we would've had to put our dogs in a kennel while we were gone.

We have traveled a lot farther many times over the years. With my two older teens being incredibly busy during their high school years, they were just as happy to relax at home and not have to sit in a van for hours at a time. Not to mention, we all preferred the comforts of home.

We attended our traditional Christmas holiday "framily" dinner too. It was a full house, and I was distracted from my thoughts. I did my best to savor the moment.

＊ ＊ ＊

It was New Year's Eve and it had been years since Mark and I had gone out to celebrate the holiday. I enjoyed spending the evening with my family. That year, especially, I was more than happy to stay home and watch one of those television shows with musical acts and a countdown to midnight. And even though I was nervous about the upcoming biopsy in January, I was ready to find some answers.

No Idea

THE END-OF-THE-YEAR FESTIVITIES WERE OVER, AND ANOTHER new year had begun. However, this particular year was already different. I started 2020 with more tests and procedures. It was only the second day of the new year and I had another medical appointment.

As that unprofessional radiologist suggested, I had a biopsy done where we found the lump. To my surprise, they also did a mammogram and another ultrasound!

First, I had to prepare for the mammogram. It was like any other routine mammogram.

After that was done, a tech led me to a small dimly lit room with a chair that leaned back. She told me to have a seat so she could do the ultrasound. Right after she finished, she left the room.

Soon after, the radiologist entered the room.

"I couldn't see anything on the mammogram," she said. "I do see something on the sonogram though. I'm just waiting for the others to join us. Where is everyone?" she said as she looked out the door.

Everyone? How many people was she expecting? A few minutes later, two other people came into the room.

As I watched the three of them stare at the sonogram, I heard the radiologist whisper something to one of her assistants.

"It's pretty big."

Next was the biopsy. Before she began the biopsy, the radiologist numbed the area where she was going to take the tissue samples. One assistant took the samples from the radiologist, and the other made notes in the chart.

"I'm putting a small metal clip inside you now," she said.

"Why do I need a clip?"

"The clip is to show where the biopsy was done. If it ends up being cancer, then the surgeon will know where to operate," she explained.

"If it's metal, then will I be able to get any MRIs done with that in me?" My eyes lit up since I don't like MRIs.

"The clip is so small that it's okay to get an MRI. Plus, your surgeon will remove the clip during your surgery."

"I see."

As far as the biopsy procedure was concerned, I won't sugarcoat it. Even though the area was numb, there was still some pain involved.

One thing that helped was to remember what it was supposed to be doing. In other words, this was how they were going to find out, for sure, if I had cancer. Putting things into perspective, not knowing for sure was a lot scarier to me than the procedure itself.

All the procedures were done in less than an hour. I never liked waiting long at a doctor's office. I mean, who does? However, that much going on in such a short amount of time was overwhelming. At least they were being thorough.

Before I left that appointment, the radiologist told me the results could take up to six days. That seemed like a quick turnaround time. I could wait six days considering I had been wondering about that lump I had noticed six weeks prior. What's another six days, right? Well, waiting those six days felt more like six months.

* * *

After talking to Mark about it first, we decided it was best to tell our teens about my potential cancer rather than wait until the day it might be confirmed. It was a quiet evening, so we decided to sit down with them and fill them in on the situation.

"I have something to tell you," I said. "I've been going to my doctor because there may be something going on with me. I found a lump here." I pointed to where the lump was. "It may be nothing, but my doctor wants to be sure. Even if it is something, like breast cancer, then it's such a common cancer that the doctors should be able to do a lot for me."

Once my husband and I shared this information with our teens, I decided to call my sister who lives out of state. Debbie is also a breast cancer survivor. I called her to get her personal perspective on how to deal with waiting for this kind of news.

"Just remember that your doctors will do whatever they have to do to get you through this," she said.

"I'm nervous because, if it is cancer, I don't know what

stage it is or if it started spreading yet."

"Try to take it one step at a time. Don't look too far ahead or it can get overwhelming."

"Thanks. I've already done some research. I'm trying not to read too much information at a time."

After that, I was a little calmer. A few days later I received that call from Dr. B confirming that I had invasive breast cancer and needed a bilateral MRI.

* * *

Two days after I had the MRI, Dr. B called again. She told me the results were in and confirmed there was no sign of cancer on the right. What a relief! At that moment, I realized that cancer is something that needs to be taken one step at a time. I promised myself that any time I started thinking too far ahead—chemo, radiation, or other treatments—I would stop and focus on the current treatment. After all, I didn't know if I would even need all those treatments for my kind of cancer, anyway.

I sat down with my husband and teens and told them the good news about the MRI results. I also told them that I may not need chemo treatments.

"I need to have other tests done and talk to other doctors before a treatment plan can be made."

* * *

Now that the bilateral MRI was done, Dr. B referred me to a surgeon. It did seem odd that we were already talking about surgery.

I made the first available appointment with the referred

surgeon, Dr. S. As the day for that appointment drew nearer, I was hearing more and more details about that new virus. I was driving my teens home from school and we caught a segment on the radio saying the first case in the United States had been reported. It was moving closer. It was very hard not to feel anxious about that.

My goal at that point was to stay focused on getting healthy. I was putting a lot of faith in my doctors and hoping the CDC—Centers for Disease Control and Prevention—could get this virus under control before it went too far.

Despite how scary things were in the world, now that I had the diagnosis and an appointment with my surgeon, I was feeling more confident about getting rid of the cancer. The way I saw it, the more hurdles I made it over, the closer I could be to living my life cancer-free.

Plus, it was hard to predict if the virus that was spreading would reach our area. And, if so, when?

* * *

Since I didn't have a primary care doctor, I searched for one and made an appointment right away. I thought it would be good to establish a relationship with this type of doctor for any general health questions as I was receiving cancer treatments.

During my appointment with my new primary care doctor, Dr. P, I asked if she could recommend a good medical oncologist. I figured I could at least get a name and be ready to contact her once I've had the surgery. With the virus spreading, I didn't want to wait too long to find the necessary doctors.

Before I left, Dr. P filled out a referral form with the

medical oncologist's name and information on it and handed it to me with a smile on her face.

"I've recommended her to other patients of mine," she reassured me.

* * *

To my surprise, I was able to make an appointment with Dr. R, the medical oncologist Dr. P recommended, right away. In fact, one of Dr. R's patients canceled so my appointment was two days before meeting my surgeon. How lucky!

The available time was not ideal for me, being so late in the day. Still, I wasn't sure when I would get another chance to meet Dr. R. So, I took the appointment. Everything seemed to be falling into place.

* * *

I went to this appointment alone since my husband needed to pick up our kids from school. The waiting room at this office was enormous with at least five people working behind the front desk. Several other patients were waiting to be seen.

While I was waiting, I heard loud chatter and laughter from a hallway adjacent to the waiting room. I could see some of the staff taking group photos of each other. It sounded like a party.

On one hand, it was nice to see coworkers getting along so well. On the other hand, I found it disturbing that they would carelessly make so much noise so close to a room with cancer patients waiting.

That appointment with Dr. R took a while. That would've

been fine if she had been helpful. Instead, she kept leaving me in the room and telling me she was trying to get the results of my past mammograms. I couldn't figure out why she wasn't able to find my results online.

"I tried calling the radiology place yesterday and nobody answered. I think maybe they weren't open because of the holiday," she claimed.

Well, two-and-a-half hours later Dr. R and I still had nothing to talk about, and she kept blaming radiology for not being available with the results. The real question was why did she wait until the day before to get the information? Plus, it seemed like she should've had access to it online anyway.

Just before I left, Dr. R suggested I get a CT scan. She even mentioned a place right across the street I could go to after my appointment. She apparently hadn't noticed the amount of time that went by during that appointment. It was already after 6 p.m., and the place she was talking about was closed for the day.

The last thing I said to her was my sister is a breast cancer survivor. She said she would also order a genetic test for me. Naturally, I left that appointment quite disappointed and was hoping that the next time I saw her she would be a lot more prepared. Strike one!

* * *

The next day I told a friend of mine what this doctor said about the radiology place where I've had mammograms in the past. She then confirmed something for me.

"I know for a fact that the radiology place *was* open on

that holiday," she said. "I had an appointment there myself that day."

* * *

It was after that when I decided to start taking notes at home right after my appointments. It was not initially with the intention of becoming a full story. I had written and self-published two children's books years ago. However, the thought of making my cancer endeavors into a story was overwhelming. My hope was that, as I was journaling, the visits with this doctor would make more sense to me somehow. That never happened.

Still, I decided to continue journaling throughout my active cancer treatments. At first, it was difficult to relive some of the moments on paper. Then it became more therapeutic than anything. I was getting over some very high hurdles.

* * *

My next appointment with Dr. R was eight days later. Dr. R worked out of two different offices. This one happened to be farther than the first one. In fact, it was twenty miles away from my home. The front desk staff scheduled this appointment time, day, and location without asking me if that would work. My thought was we needed to get started on things sooner than later, so I didn't argue.

That time Mark went with me. We were lucky enough to get our kids to school on time and then head straight to my appointment. We arrived about ten minutes early.

I overheard a nurse ask if Dr. R had arrived yet. That wasn't a good sign. She finally entered the building thirty minutes after my scheduled appointment time. I was really hoping she was at least more prepared for this appointment.

Since she said she would order the genetic test, and I was able to get the CT the day after my first appointment with her, I figured that should be enough time for her to get the genetic test results and review the CT scans. Well, I figured it wrong. Once again, she did not have much information.

She could only tell us some of the CT scan results, which my surgeon had already filled us in on completely the week before. She did not have the genetic test results.

I'm not saying that she had complete control over getting results from other places. My question is, what was the point of going that far to an appointment if she didn't have much to say? It wasn't any better than the first visit with her. Strike two!

* * *

About five weeks later I was at yet another appointment with Dr. R. Before then, I was able to meet my surgeon, have the surgery, and see my new primary care doctor again.

This time Dr. R had my genetic test results. Hooray! I was hoping that meant she had a treatment plan for me. Not knowing what it took to create a treatment plan, I asked her what was supposed to happen next.

"I was looking to see if you had an Oncotype test done and can't find it anywhere!" Her eyes darted back and forth across her computer screen.

An Oncotype test? That was the first time I had heard of that test. She never mentioned it at my first two appointments. As my husband and I, and an intern, watched Dr. R stare at her computer waiting for test results, I was thinking it was time to find another doctor. Later, I found some vital information online that Dr. R should have known. From Genomic Health Inc.:

> It is important that your doctor requests the Oncotype DX Breast Recurrence Score test before you start any treatment since the test results are intended for use in guiding the selection of your treatment. Most test results are available within 7 to 10 days from the date your tumor sample is received by the Genomic Health laboratory.

The appointment continued with Dr. R consistently leaving the room and coming back saying that she was trying to get info on my Oncotype test. You know, the one most likely not ordered.

I think her intern was starting to feel sorry for us. The intern offered to get us something to drink. We politely declined. I just wanted to get out of there.

"I just chewed out your surgeon!" Dr. R said as she strutted back into the room once again. "She should've ordered the Oncotype test for you!"

That struck a nerve with me because I have the utmost respect for my surgeon. Why was that the first time it was even mentioned? Plus, that was the third time she was blaming someone else for her not having the proper information to build my treatment plan.

Wasn't she supposed to take the lead on my case? It also seemed odd that she wasn't even interested in checking me physically considering I had my surgery a few weeks before that appointment. What was going on with her?

Once again, I had an appointment with little information and without knowing what to do next. Then, Dr. R said something that finally drove me to find another medical oncologist.

"So, you and I will be seeing each other for the next ten years."

"Okay," I said.

That was about all I *could* say even though I knew there was no way I would be going back to her again. Strike three! She's out of there!

* * *

Only two days after I initially met Dr. R I had my first appointment with Dr. S. She was the wonderful surgeon Dr. B had referred to me. I trusted Dr. B knew who the best surgeon would be for me. I was so glad I did too.

Mark and I arrived about fifteen minutes early for my appointment. The waiting room had maybe twenty seats lined along the walls. One other patient was in there sitting across the room from us.

So far, this was like any other doctor's appointment I've had over the years. It really didn't seem like I was there for anything serious.

In a corner nearby there was a table with brochures filled with information on free workshops for cancer patients. I glanced through a couple of them then brought them back to my seat. Suddenly this seemed real.

"Ms. Ormsby, you can follow me now."

Mark stayed in the waiting room while I was escorted back

to a small room with a reclining seat in it. It was a little cool in there, but it was still comfortable enough.

Before we discussed the results of the tests I had over several weeks, Dr. S checked me with the ultrasound. She also asked if her intern could check me too.

"Yes, of course, she can. The more practice the better she'll be, right?"

The ultrasounds were done, and Dr. S invited Mark and me to her office to discuss the results of the tests. I had no idea how involved breast cancer could be!

As she drew pictures and labeled them to describe my cancer and surgery in detail, it became quite clear to me that I had found the right surgeon.

"First of all, your CT scan looked fine. There didn't seem to be any signs of cancer anywhere else."

"Great!" My shoulders lowered a bit.

Interesting that Dr. S was able to get the CT results the day after I had the test. What a difference between her and Dr. R. I was already feeling more at ease.

"You have the best-case scenario. Your cancer is stage two, grade two. So, it was caught early. You're also ER positive, PR positive, and HER2 negative," Dr. S continued.

I had heard of cancer stages before, but not any of the other factors. She had an incredible way of explaining things. She had the results and was talking about everything my cancer involved. That was such a nice change of pace.

"ER means estrogen receptor and PR stands for progesterone receptor," she said. "Since they were both positive, your cancer cells were growing in response to them. When cancer cells are HER2 negative that means the cells have a low level of the protein human epidermal growth factor receptor 2. That means the cells will grow slower and divide less, which is what you want."

"So, why are ER positive and PR positive good things?" I asked. "Usually, positive results on a medical test are not good."

"When a person is ER and PR positive that means they can get hormone therapy to slow down or maybe even prevent those cancer cells from coming back," she explained.

She told me about my surgery options. While I appreciated having choices, however, it wasn't an easy decision. As she wrote the choices down on paper, she explained them to me in simple terms.

"You can get a lumpectomy and radiation, or you can have a mastectomy, and possibly reconstruction, with radiation. Either one will also include a sentinel node biopsy," she said.

"Okay, so how do I decide what type of surgery I need? I mean, of course, I would prefer the less-aggressive one. Still, how do I know if that's enough for my cancer?"

"I wouldn't be offering a lumpectomy if I didn't think that was enough for your type of cancer. Plus, since it was caught early, you can go with the less-aggressive surgery."

"A lumpectomy it is then. How is that done?"

I couldn't believe I was asking those questions. Sometimes I can get weak in the knees hearing medical jargon. I wanted to be as informed as possible, though.

"The tumor and some surrounding tissue will be removed to be sure I get everything that may be cancer," she explained. "I'll also remove a few nearby lymph nodes and send them to the lab to see if it has spread at all."

As scary as cancer can be, it was amazing how the right doctor could make me feel so much better. And she hadn't even performed the surgery yet!

Before we left, someone in her office scheduled me for the surgery. Mark and I walked out of that office feeling reassured. Everything was going to be all right.

* * *

My surgery was on February 18. My stomach was empty. I had been fasting since midnight. We arrived at 8 a.m. and waited for about an hour.

"Ms. Ormsby?" a nurse called.

She took me to a room the size of a small closet to change out of my clothes and into a full-length fabric gown.

"Put this robe on because we'll be cutting through the waiting room," the nurse said.

Boy, she was not kidding. The walk to radiology was something I'll never forget. I was wearing a hospital gown for the surgery and, to my surprise, I was walking through a very full waiting room!

I ended up in a room with other women who were waiting for their mammograms. I was the only one dressed for surgery, which was a little uncomfortable.

I imagined they were all there to see if they were still healthy. I was there because I knew I had cancer. Then I wondered why I was in that room with the others.

It was in a nearby room that I was prepped for my surgery. I had a blue dye injected into the area around my tumor. Then the dye was supposed to travel to the nearby lymph nodes to help my surgeon find and remove them. It was both fascinating and frightening.

My surgery was about two hours behind schedule. As I was waiting for my turn, I grew more and more concerned about my blood sugar. I had been fasting for almost ten hours and now my surgery was delayed. My husband was politely eating his lunch outside my room since I couldn't eat. I called the nurse.

"I have type II diabetes and haven't eaten for some time. Is it possible to have my blood sugar checked?" I wasn't sure she would've been willing to do that.

"Of course, we can!" she said with a smile.

To my surprise, my blood sugar was around 140, so I was fine for the time being.

The surgery was done and it was a big success! The anesthesia started to wear off, and I slowly awakened to find myself with a bandage tightly wrapped around my chest like a mummy. A nurse was standing next to my bed smiling at me.

"You need to keep those bandages on for the next forty-eight hours," she said. "Your doctor prescribed pain medicine for you because you'll feel more pain once the anesthesia completely wears off."

I was still out of it, but I remember that Mark approached my bed and smiled. "Welcome back," he said.

"Hi."

That's about all I could say for the time being. I was concerned about the bandages around me. I could breathe just fine if I didn't try to take any deep breaths. I started to get dressed but needed Mark to help me put my shirt on over the bulky bandages. Then we headed home.

As soon as Mark and I walked into our home our two oldest were standing there with t-shirts on that had a pink ribbon and said, "Child of a Warrior." That made my day. That was exactly the kind of support I needed!

* * *

Now that I was home again, Mark ran out to get my prescription pain medicine. Dr. S prescribed Percocet, which has acetaminophen and oxycodone. At first, I was leery of taking it. Her instructions were to take it every six hours if needed. Boy, did I ever need it!

I continued taking it every six hours for the next three days. I didn't like how it made me feel loopy, but at least I was in less pain. It also made me drowsy. It was such a strong medicine that I couldn't leave my house for the first few days after my surgery.

Each time I took the Percocet, around four hours after, the pain would start to increase again. Around the fifth hour, it was almost unbearable! I distracted myself until the sixth hour arrived. I watched television, played games on my phone, or just talked to Mark since he stayed home to help me through the first few days.

When it was time to remove the bandages, I made sure to do it about fifteen minutes after I took a Percocet. That way, if the pain was much stronger without the bandages initially, I'd be prepared.

Three days after my surgery, the Percocet was gone. Even

though I was tempted to ask for more, I decided to try over-the-counter pain medicine instead. It worked better than I thought it would. I was so relieved that I was no longer taking an opioid, too. I knew how addictive those could be. It helped that I wasn't doing as much at home as I usually did.

* * *

One way I did less was to accept meals from other families. Ruth, a pastor at Cedar Ridge, was kind enough to offer a sign-up for other church families to prepare meals for my family during my recovery time. She was the first to bring a meal to us, and it was soon after my surgery. What we didn't know was just how much food we would get! Each meal covered at least a few evenings of dinner for my family.

In addition to the church family meals, a few neighbors brought dishes over to us. In fact, the Sunday after my surgery we received three large family meals before the day was done! It was uplifting to see how many people cared about us.

My good friend Trica and her adult children brought over a purple hand-knitted prayer shawl from her church. It was made specifically for people dealing with something difficult. The tag on it read, "Made for you with Love." To this day, I like covering up with it, especially whenever I'm feeling discouraged.

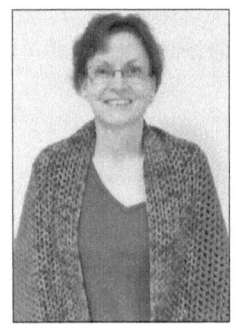

Support shawl.
Photo by Mark Ormsby

A close and longtime friend, Julie, sent a big care package with breast cancer awareness items and a few extra "supportive friend" goodies.

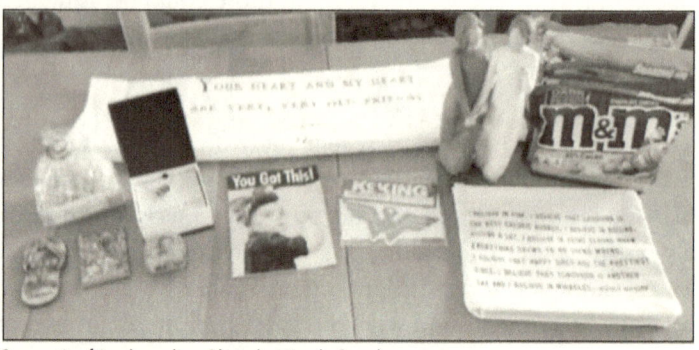

Supportive friend goodies. *Photo by Wendy Ormsby*

The compassion did not stop there. My sister-in-law, Anne, sent many items to me for encouragement and support. She also called me often as I was going through chemotherapy and radiation, which made my treatments more bearable. I was grateful for that.

My husband and two older teens were quite supportive throughout my active treatments. I would get occasional calls from my parents, two brothers, and my sister. I also had many other friends who were checking on me often to see how I was feeling during all my different treatments.

My dear friend Bev had even given me advice on how to handle those claustrophobic MRI machines. "I like to go through the alphabet and choose a person who starts with each letter then pray for them. It's a nice way to pass the time," she said.

She's so sweet!

Some of those friendships started as recently as a couple of years ago. However, my friendship with Julie has been almost a lifetime so far. We have been the closest of friends for over forty years now.

Whenever I started to feel stressed, I'd call or text Julie. She would modestly give me her take on my situation and did so with compassion and an open mind and without any expectations. To me, that is the very definition of a friend.

* * *

Not long after my surgery, I had a follow-up with Dr. S. My husband came with me to this appointment too.

"Once I removed your tumor it measured smaller than we had originally thought it was," she said. "So, it was stage one, not stage two. And there were cancer cells in one of the three nearby lymph nodes I removed. That's okay because now they'll know where to focus during radiation treatments."

I was so glad the tumor was smaller than they had originally thought. However, it was distressing to hear about the cancer in one of the lymph nodes. Despite that, I still had some relief from the idea of radiation taking care of it.

"Um, I know I'm still wearing a gown," I said. "Can I have a hug?"

"Yes, you look like you could use a hug," Dr. S said with a smile.

Only two-and-a-half weeks later, the first COVID-19 positive cases were confirmed in our immediate area. I was so grateful for my surgeon.

- 4 -

Still Searching

MY SURGERY WAS DONE, AND I FELT GOOD ABOUT MY PROGRESS so far. However, I was still looking for a good medical oncologist. I also had a noticeable amount of pain and stiffness in my left shoulder from the surgery. Plus, I was in search of a radiation oncologist. That was a lot to think about. It helped to keep in mind my goal of being "cancer-free."

A few weeks after my surgery I met with Dr. F, my radiation oncologist, for the first time. I still had a lot of pain and stiffness in my left shoulder. Before meeting Dr. F, Nurse M took my vitals and made sure my medical history was updated. She was quite friendly. In fact, she was so friendly that I was comfortable telling her about my shoulder problem.

"Hi, Ms. Ormsby. How are you feeling today?"

"My left shoulder still has a lot of pain and stiffness. I can barely lift my arm up to reach anything."

"I know a great physical therapist who works with breast cancer patients!" she offered. "Her office is right next door."

She gave me the contact information of the physical therapist. That was a pleasant surprise, considering she wasn't even my doctor! Nurse M then took me to meet my radiation oncologist.

I mentioned my shoulder problem to Dr. F too, and she said to start PT as soon as possible. I needed my range of motion back for radiation therapy since I would have to raise my arms while I was lying on the table for treatments.

We also talked about how radiation would work. It was a long appointment but well worth it. She was very good at explaining what was involved in radiation treatments. I looked online ahead of time to gather the best possible questions I could for this appointment.

"How will radiation therapy affect my risk of local breast cancer recurrence, metastasis, or a new breast cancer?" I asked.

"It will lower your risk, especially for positive node cancer. It will include locoregional therapy so the breast and lymph nodes both receive treatment."

"How long will each session take and how many sessions will I need?" I continued.

"Each entire session will be about twenty minutes long and it will be daily, Monday through Friday, for four to six weeks," she explained.

"What side effects should I expect from radiation?"

"Short-term side effects might be mild fatigue and a skin reaction. Long-term effects may be chest wall tightness, possible lung irritation, fever, and your breast tissue may be about 5% smaller after radiation is done."

Oddly enough, guess which one of those stood out in my

mind? I don't mind the surgical scar; it reminds me that I survived something really scary. However, I didn't know radiation could shrink the tissue. At least it was caught early.

As Dr. F and I were still talking in her office something dawned on me. With COVID-19 spreading throughout the United States, I was wondering if I would be able to start radiation. I wasn't sure if their office would even stay open. That was obviously something I couldn't do at home.

"So, will I be able to start radiation even though there's a pandemic?"

"If you end up needing chemo, you may not be able to start that right away because of the pandemic. It weakens your immune system. As far as starting with radiation, we may have to close our office. You can possibly start with hormone therapy since you can do that at home. That's something you can ask your medical oncologist."

"Oh boy. Let's hope people take this seriously enough so this pandemic will be over sooner than later," I said. "At least I've had my surgery. That's good."

Turned out it really *was* good. Less than two weeks later, nonessential businesses in my area were starting to close. Health care services were also affected by the pandemic. Things were changing quickly. From the Ambulatory Surgery Center Association and ASCA Foundation:

...an additional executive order on March 16 related to health care services: the order includes a provision authorizing the Secretary of Health to, "take actions to control, restrict, and regulate the use of health care facilities for the performance of elective medical procedures, as neces-

sary to respond to the catastrophic health emergency." On March 23 the Maryland Department of Health released a Directive and Order Regarding Various Healthcare Matters. The directive provides that, "pursuant to the Executive Order of March 16 relating to various health care matters... all licensed hospitals, ambulatory surgical centers, and all other licensed health care facilities shall cease all elective and non-urgent medical procedures effective at 5 p.m., Tuesday, March 24, 2020, and not provide any such procedures for the duration of the catastrophic health emergency."

The last thing Dr. F and I discussed was the fact that I still needed a new medical oncologist. I told her about one I found online. I was impressed with her bio and thought she might be a good oncologist for me. I also mentioned that the oncologist happened to be upstairs in the same building.

"Well, it's not too late if you want to go upstairs to make an appointment with her," she suggested.

* * *

I excitedly walked out of the radiation center and went directly upstairs to make an appointment. It wasn't as easy as I was hoping it would be. It was incredibly busy in that office. Keeping in mind COVID was in my area, I was suddenly more nervous than ever at a medical office. Since I was already there, I went ahead and approached the front desk.

"Hi. I'd like to make an appointment with a doctor here."

"May I have your name, please?"

As soon as I gave her my name things started getting more difficult. I just wanted someone qualified to help me. She didn't even need to have a great bedside manner at this point.

"You already have a doctor in this practice, ma'am."

"I know. I would like a different one, please."

"We can probably do that," she said. "We'll have to ask your current doctor first."

How awkward it would be to let Dr. R know that I was leaving her for one of her colleagues. Then I realized something: Who cares? If she wasn't going to take care of me, I needed to find someone who would.

"That's fine," I replied.

"Okay. I'll call your current doctor right now so you can make an appointment with your new doctor."

I had a feeling that wouldn't be simple. As I was watching and waiting for her to talk to Dr. R on the phone, I noticed there was no phone conversation. The woman hung up the phone and started talking to me again.

"She isn't available to speak with right now."

Despite not getting Dr. R's permission, I was still able to schedule an appointment with Dr. C. I was set to meet my new medical oncologist in two weeks and could hardly wait. Finally, I had a qualified medical oncologist.

* * *

As Dr. F said, I needed physical therapy, so I'd be ready for radiation. I took Nurse M's advice and made an appointment with the physical therapist near the radiation center six days later.

COVID cases were rising in our area. More and more people were wearing masks everywhere. Still, I had to do something about my shoulder before radiation treatments started.

"So, tell me what's going on with you," my physical therapist, Dr. M, said through her mask.

"I recently had a lumpectomy and have had pain and stiffness in my left shoulder," I explained.

"Okay, then. Let's see what exercises would work best for you. Show me how high you can lift your arm."

"Not very high at all." I winced as I struggled to raise my left arm. "I've had to use my right arm more since I can't bring my left arm high enough. Among other things, it makes washing my hair and pulling things down from the kitchen cabinets a lot more difficult."

She showed me some stretches that could help loosen the muscles in my chest, left shoulder, and arm. I tried them before I left. Unfortunately, I didn't get very far, but at least I had a plan.

"If you need anything while you're at home, like harder or different exercises, please let me know," she said. "I'll give you a printout of what we did today to take home with you. And I'm going to give you my personal email in case our clinic closes soon because of the pandemic."

Luckily, I had an understanding and compassionate physical therapist. We agreed after the evaluation that I could do my exercises at home where it should be safer during the pandemic. I was really hoping those stretches would do the trick.

I have been a very active person over the years. Unfortunately, I've also had many reasons to need physical therapy. I've had a few good physical therapists who really did help me recover from my injuries.

Dr. M had such a delicate way of dealing with my situation that I knew I would be okay soon enough. About three weeks after I started physical therapy, I was already regaining full range of motion in my left arm and feeling much better.

* * *

One of my biggest concerns was not being up to a healthy weight when I started my cancer treatments. I've read that some cancer patients lose weight and others gain throughout their treatments. It would've been okay if I had gained a few pounds.

So, I walked my dogs when the weather was nice. Walking did help me work up an appetite but only a little. Believe me, I never thought that would be a problem at that stage of my life.

* * *

When a person has cancer treatments to think about, it can be challenging to remember annual appointments, especially during a pandemic. Nevertheless, I was due for my annual exam with my gynecologist.

Since we had positive cases of COVID in our area, her office had already started implementing some guidelines. Their office was not mandating wearing masks in public yet, but I did have the choice to wait in my vehicle and they would call me when it was my turn.

While I was with my doctor, I mentioned my appointment coming up with Dr. C. She seemed happy for me and referred to Dr. C as the "guru of breast cancer." I was so glad to hear that.

* * *

Now that I had a new medical oncologist, I was ready to start figuring out a plan. It was late March, and I was meeting Dr. C at a virtual appointment. It was great to have a second chance after what happened with the first doctor. It was great, at least, until the appointment started.

"Hi. How are you?" Dr. C asked.

"I'm ready for a plan!"

"Okay, well, let's see…What tests have you done?"

"My most recent one was the Oncotype test."

Hoping history was not repeating itself, I wondered why she was asking me about the tests. Fortunately, I called ahead and was able to get the results of the Oncotype test. After all, it was supposed to have been ordered almost three weeks prior to that appointment. If Dr. C didn't have the results, at least I would.

"What was your score on the Oncotype test?" Her question and blank expression confirmed my thoughts about her. She was not at all prepared for this visit.

"My score was 20." My voice grew quieter.

As the appointment continued, she kept referring to the fact that *I* was telling her the test result. Somehow, she didn't see anything wrong with that. I was dumbfounded. I couldn't understand why a doctor who had been in that field for so long would be talking like that.

"So, what does that score mean to you?" I asked.

"Well, your score was 20 because you told me it was. That's a moderate score."

I already knew it was a "moderate" score. As we were talking, she kept trying to look information up online about the Oncotype test. Was this a new test for her?

Unlike her, I did my homework. Before my appointment, I did some research on that test, so I had an idea about what the score meant. I wanted to know what it meant to her though.

She was the doctor. I was the patient.

"There are three scores you can have," she said. "High, moderate, and low."

"So, what does my moderate score mean as far as my treatment plan?"

What was happening? Was I asking the wrong questions? Instead of deciding on a plan from that test score, she came up with another test for me.

"I'm going to order a MammaPrint test for you."

"A what?"

"This test only has high and low scores. That way there won't be any gray areas. It tells what your risk of recurrence would be. I have a feeling your score will be low." She suddenly sounded confident.

So, I was back to waiting for another test result and hoping Dr. C ordered it like she said she would. At least, maybe, that would help her figure out a plan once and for all.

* * *

It was early spring 2020 and my weight was only in the double digits. I just couldn't get my appetite back. I don't remember the last time I weighed so little. I had lost thirty pounds over the previous two years. My tooth problem was resolved, but I still couldn't eat much. If I did end up needing chemo and lost weight during treatments, I desperately needed to gain some weight back before then.

* * *

Before my active cancer treatments started, my friend Shobha from church connected me with her friend Colleen, who had many personal experiences with cancer. I called Colleen to get her insight on cancer. We talked for over three hours, and it was one of the most memorable phone conversations I've ever had!

She was so open about her many cancer recurrences over a seventeen-year span. When she spoke, she did so in such a calm manner that it made me feel like everything was going to be okay. I couldn't imagine how one person could go through all that, over and over, and still be so pleasant toward others.

That memorable phone call with her really put my cancer into perspective. She continued to support me through encouraging text messages whenever she was able to since she was also going through cancer treatments.

* * *

Still waiting to hear back from Dr. C, I called to see if she had ordered the MammaPrint test for me since we were counting on that to help decide on chemotherapy. The MammaPrint test had been ordered. The results were not in yet.

A few days later, I received a phone call from Dr. C.

"Hello, is this Ms. Ormsby? I have the results of your MammaPrint test. You're in the high-risk category," she said.

My heart sank.

"I thought you figured I would be *low* risk."

"I did, but you're not."

"So, now what? Does that mean I'll need chemo after all?"

"*You* know what it means."

"No, I don't know." My jaw clenched. That was not a time for more noncommittal responses. It was time to decide on a plan. I had finally had enough.

"Look," I said. "First, you didn't have any information ready at my appointment with you. Then, even after I gave you some information, you did nothing with it. Then, you wanted to order another test. And now, you're still not telling me what to do."

"Well! I have been doing this job for thirty-one years. But if you want to find another medical oncologist, then go right ahead!"

"As a matter of fact, I do."

* * *

The search for a good medical oncologist continued. It didn't seem like that should have been so challenging in the Washington, D.C. area. There were plenty of doctors in so many fields nearby. Why *was* that so difficult, anyway? I had already given that practice two chances and they were 0 for 2. It was time to look somewhere else.

Since I was building my care with more and more Johns Hopkins doctors, why not find a medical oncologist through them? Along with Colleen, I spoke with another friend who had a relative with breast cancer, with my radiation oncologist, and with yet another friend's neighbor who was a medical oncologist. The neighbor used to work at a nearby hospital but switched to doing more of the research end of things.

After speaking with everyone, I noticed there was one thing they all had in common. They all highly recommended the same practice! And, it was not only the same practice, but I kept hearing the same two doctor's names. I was really hoping that was a sign of something great to come!

I don't think there was ever a time in my life when I wanted this third time to be a charm more than ever. Unlike the first time I switched doctors, I did not notify my current medical oncologist. It was mostly because I wanted to make sure I had a new and capable doctor to replace her first. Besides, I had already made it clear over the phone that I was not happy with how things were going.

I contacted the office with the two highly recommended doctors. I've never been comfortable cold calling anywhere, especially a doctor's office. I guess maybe it's because most offices are busy, and I feel like I should talk fast to get my message across to them. That call was a real emotional rollercoaster.

"Hello. May I help you?" The receptionist had a pleasant voice.

"Yes, hi. I'd like to make an appointment with one of your medical oncologists."

"Do you have a referral from your primary care doctor?"

"Uh, no. I do not. What I'm trying to do is change doctors."

"Change doctors?"

"Yes. Technically, I already have a medical oncologist. I'd like to see someone else—"

"I'm sorry, ma'am. You can't get a second opinion from another Johns Hopkins doctor."

"But I don't think my current doctor works for Johns Hopkins."

"And because of the pandemic, we have been limiting the

number of appointments and trying to avoid any unnecessary changes with doctors."

At that point in the conversation, many thoughts were coming to me. Would I have to stay with Dr. C even though she was so exhausting? I knew Dr. R and Dr. C were not Johns Hopkins doctors. How was I able to get a second opinion when I switched from Dr. R to Dr. C? Then again, that was hardly an opinion.

Then, perhaps in desperation, I chose to do something I wouldn't ordinarily be comfortable doing. I was brutally honest. I could not see myself staying with either of the first two doctors for the next ten years. What I said to her next was really referring to both medical oncologists that I had seen.

"All right, here's the thing. I haven't really *had* an opinion yet. I've had a very hard time getting anywhere with the medical oncologist I currently have. Cancer is stressful enough without having a doctor who is not doing her job. She's never prepared and doesn't seem to know what to do about my cancer. Not to mention, she's quite full of herself!"

Okay, so maybe that last statement was unnecessary. Unfortunately, it was true. And as I said, I was desperate. It was a combination of getting some pent-up feelings off my chest and hopefully getting an appointment with a medical oncologist who would *help* me. No matter what the reason was, I was so glad I said those things. She asked me for information on Dr. C.

I told her my doctor's full name and where she worked. I couldn't believe what happened next. The situation started changing. She was talking like she knew her.

"Do you know my current doctor?" I asked.

"No, but many people have come here from her office because she was no help to them either. I'm going to set up an appointment for you with one of our doctors. Did you have a particular one in mind?"

I was not alone. What an incredible feeling.

Things were suddenly looking up for me. What were the odds of me getting one of the two that my friends had highly recommended? The conversation ended with her scheduling me with one of the recommended doctors. Amazing!

* * *

It was May 5, 2020, and that year my celebration of Cinco de Mayo was already quite nontraditional. I was sitting in front of my computer at home anxiously waiting for my first virtual appointment with my newest medical oncologist. This time I was more prepared for my appointment. I searched through sites looking for information about the benefits of chemo. I was ready to ask detailed questions about my type of cancer.

"Good morning, how are you feeling?" Dr. N asked.

"I'm feeling okay. Still wondering if I'll need chemo or not."

"We're going to figure that out today," she said. "Do you have any questions for me to start?"

"What is the best way to interpret my test results in order to get the best treatment plan?"

"We will look at your cancer stage and the size and grade of your tumor. Your intermediate Oncotype score of 20 means the benefit of chemo cannot be excluded."

"Would you recommend chemo for me then?" I asked.

"Since the MammaPrint test results were high risk, chemo may be beneficial. You also had cancer cells in one of your sentinel lymph nodes. There are potential side effects to chemo, so we need to figure out if the benefits outweigh the side effects."

Incredible! She was answering all my questions and putting so much thought into my treatment plan! Hard to believe she had the same information as the last doctor who didn't help me at all. Some may see this differently, but the next thing she said about chemo convinced me that she was the one for me.

"If it's okay with you, I'd like to consult with my colleagues at Johns Hopkins before we fully commit to it. If you don't hear from me by Friday, then email me."

"That's fine with me! Thanks for asking." I was breathing easier.

Dr. N called me the next day to tell me what she and her colleagues had decided. She said there was a consensus that I should have chemo. There were just too many gray areas, and it was better to err on the side of caution. We had a plan at last! Of course, after that news, I had more questions.

"How aggressive do you think my chemo will need to be?"

"Less aggressive than some since you are ER positive and endocrine therapy will help you too. You'll need four sessions, instead of eight, with only two drugs," she clarified.

"Considering we're in the middle of a pandemic, when should I start the chemo treatments?"

"You can start chemo soon. We'll take all the necessary universal precautions."

"Can my chemo be given as a pill instead?"

"No. You'll need to come in and have it done intravenously.

You'll also have bloodwork done before each session. Your treatments will be every three weeks with a total of four sessions over twelve weeks. I'll send more info to you on the chemo treatments."

That all sounded overwhelming. At least I had a medical oncologist who knew what she was talking about. In fact, it sounded like Dr. N had been in the field for years. In my opinion, that's how a medical oncologist *should* sound.

"What can be the side effects of this chemo?" I asked.

"Hair loss, fatigue, and lowering of your blood count, which can weaken your immune system. The first round of chemo usually has the worst nausea along with numbness and tingling in the fingers. Then it should get better after that."

"What should I avoid during treatment?" "Just make sure you keep 'social distancing' because of COVID-19."

What a different feeling than with Dr. C!

* * *

My first face-to-face appointment with her was only a week later. At that appointment, she introduced me to her nurse practitioner who was across the room from us. Dr. N said that sometimes I would be seen by her instead. She asked Nurse L if she thought I would need a port or if my veins were good enough for the IV.

"I can see her veins from here!" Nurse L said with a smile.

"Then I guess you're fine with just the IV," Dr. N confirmed.

Dr. N gave me a physical and I had bloodwork done. The physical and bloodwork became the routine before each round of chemo.

As intimidating as the upcoming months seemed, I was ready to take the next step toward recovery. I was also keeping in mind that it was best to take things one step at a time and not think too far ahead. The surgery was done, and chemo was next.

* * *

It was a relief to finally have a complete team of doctors for my cancer care. The road to finding those doctors had some big bumps along the way, so I really appreciated the extra inspiration to keep me going. Maybe it wouldn't work for everyone, but hearing fighting words like "battle," "beat," and "Warrior" from friends and loved ones helped me tremendously.

I texted Colleen and asked her an important question. She had had so much to deal with over the years.

"May I ask how you keep your spirits up?"

"Good question," she replied. "Being a natural 'glass half empty' type of person, working on gratitude has been a major factor. I don't mean being thankful for cancer but thankful for beauty, relationships, all the material things I have, etc. I also think it's important to laugh and have a sense of humor. Most importantly, it's important to live in the moment."

- 5 -

A Full-Time Job

BEFORE I COULD START CHEMO, I NEEDED TO ANSWER COVID-19 questions online. The number of positive cases was so high in New York that I was asked if I had recently traveled there. Thankfully, no. Another question was, had I recently come in close contact with anyone who tested positive for COVID? It was hard to know that for sure. To my knowledge, I hadn't. Then they asked me if I had any COVID symptoms. Again, thankfully, no.

A couple of days later I had my first round of chemo. Mark offered to drive me to my appointment. He just wanted it to be less stressful for me. I was so grateful for the fact that he was working from home due to the pandemic.

On our way to the hospital, I pictured myself in an over-stuffed reclining chair in a big room full of people. That's how I've always seen chemotherapy shown in movies. I was hoping to meet other cancer patients so we could commiserate with each other.

When I walked into the hospital for the first round, I had to stop at a table near the entrance. A man sitting there asked me the same COVID questions I filled out online. That was confusing. Fortunately, my answers hadn't changed so he let me continue toward the oncology unit.

* * *

I entered the oncology unit and noticed several people sitting to my right in an open room the size of living and dining rooms combined. Some of the chairs had tape across them so patients sat no closer than six feet from each other. The lines for checking in had big round stickers on the floor showing where to stand so you were six feet from the person in front of you. It was my turn, so I approached the woman at the desk who was behind plexiglass.

"Hi. I'm—"

"Good morning. Please stay back on the first sticker. I'll be able to hear you from there."

With my face a darker pink, I took a few steps back to stand on the sticker. "I'm here for my chemo treatment."

"Okay. Have you recently traveled to New York?"

"No, I haven't."

"Have you been in close contact with anyone who tested positive for COVID-19 in the last fourteen days?"

"No, I haven't."

"Do you currently have a fever or chills, cough, shortness of breath, fatigue, nausea or vomiting, diarrhea, or muscle or body aches?"

"No, I do not."

This was the third time I was answering questions concerning COVID. I tried not to roll my eyes. At least they were being careful.

I had already looked up the potential side effects of chemo so I would be prepared. COVID symptoms sounded a lot like some of the chemo side effects. Once my first treatment was over, I hoped I would be able to tell the difference.

* * *

It wasn't long at all before someone called my name. A woman escorted me down a few hallways and into a tiny room. It had one vinyl reclining chair in the corner, a small table on wheels, and a television set across from the chair on the wall. I was surprised that many items could fit in there. The room smelled like rubbing alcohol from the COVID cleaning just before I had arrived.

"Your nurse will be with you soon to start your treatment," she said.

The nurse for my first round of chemo, Nurse C, was attentive and told me some of the physical changes that might occur from the chemo. Of course, I was hoping most of the things she mentioned would not actually happen.

"You will lose your hair with this chemo, especially since your hair is so fine already."

"The color and shape of your nails will change."

"And you will most likely feel very tired and maybe nauseous early on as your body gets used to the drugs."

Even though I had done my research on chemo side effects, and Nurse C was clear about what could happen, there was no way to fully prepare myself mentally. Attach a pandemic to that and it was even more disconcerting.

"We're going to start you off with some saline," she continued. "Then, we'll add your first of two chemo meds."

"Okay. I'm ready."

Was I ready? It was hard to know. Until that day, I didn't think about how it might feel having chemo meds running through my veins.

"Everything should take about two hours," she said. "The saline is going, and I'll be back a little later to start your first chemo med."

Since I was wearing a mask the entire time, it was comforting to know that I wouldn't be there all day.

As I waited for the saline drip to be done, I tried to make myself more comfortable in the sticky vinyl chair. The television was off, and I could hear muffled conversations between the nurses outside my room. It was quieter than I expected it to be.

After the saline had been running for a while, Nurse C came in covered from head to toe in protective gear to start me on my first chemo medicine.

"I have to wear a mask, a shield, and a gown in case any of your chemo medicine spills while I'm setting it up for you. There, now you're getting your first chemo med," she confirmed.

It was scary that she needed so much protection from the medicine that was about to go through my veins. Of course, it was also going to help get rid of my cancer. That's what I had to keep in mind.

I know it was bad timing on my part, but it seemed like the saline kicked in soon after she started the first chemo drug. I noticed that my medicines were hooked onto a pole on wheels. Before Nurse C left the room, I asked her if I could use the restroom.

"Sure. I'll just unplug the machine from the wall, and you can roll the pole into the bathroom with you."

Simple enough.

She unplugged the machine and headed out my door. I slowly walked a few feet to the doorway of my room. My nurse was watching me from across the nurse's station. I started feeling like I was almost floating.

The rush of heat was overwhelming, and the muffled conversations were gone. It was as if I was entering a dark tunnel. I leaned against the frame of my door.

"Are you okay?" she asked.

"Not...really," I struggled to say through my mask.

Nurse C was back in my room within seconds. She told me to have a seat. The next thing I knew, four other people were gathering near my room to help. My chair was now in its upright position. The quietness was gone.

There was no way we were all six feet apart. For the first time since the pandemic started, I did not care. Nurse C was talking to me, but I wasn't sure why there were other people there.

"What's happening?" I tried not to panic.

"You're having an allergic reaction to the chemo med," said Nurse C.

Some of the staff outside my room approached me. There

was so much commotion and none of it made any sense. Nurse J introduced herself and said she was the nurse who handled emergencies.

I need an "emergency" nurse?!

"My back! I feel shooting pains in my lower back! And my heart feels like it's beating out of my chest!"

A nurse pulled my face mask off so she could give me oxygen. I wasn't sure I needed it, but I was not about to argue with anyone trying to help me. I sat there and wondered what was next. What a surreal moment.

"We're giving you some Benadryl through your IV now to counteract your allergic reaction," said Nurse J.

At first, the Benadryl itself was causing a bad reaction. I started feeling more overheated, dizzier, and extremely sleepy. A few minutes later, everything calmed down.

Everyone except Nurse C left my room. She waited to make sure the Benadryl was working then said she would be back soon to continue my chemo treatment.

"Wait, you mean I'll be getting the same medicine again?"

"Yes. I'll speak to your doctor first to make sure. Of course, it should be fine now that you've had the Benadryl."

Oh boy. I was really hoping she was right.

Nurse C came back a few minutes later.

"Your doctor told me to use a slow drip in addition to the 25 milligrams of Benadryl just in case," she said.

"I am so nervous trying this chemo medicine again."

"Don't worry. You'll be fine this time."

"Can you stay for a few minutes once you start the medicine?" I asked.

It took five hours from start to finish. That was more than twice the time they had expected. Thankfully, everything ran smoother once I had Benadryl.

* * *

I returned the next day for a white blood cell injection to boost my immune system. Although it would take a couple of weeks to kick in, I was grateful for that injection, especially during a pandemic.

After the nurse gave me the injection, she handed me information on how to give myself the other three injections at home so I wouldn't have to come in as often during a pandemic. I had never done anything like that before, but I seriously considered it.

* * *

I was back home and there was a pleasant surprise that evening. I knew I would lose my hair with this chemo. Rather than watching long strands fall out in the shower, I thought it would be less traumatic if I started with much shorter hair. I asked my husband to cut it short for me. What I didn't know was how liberating it would be! I've never had wash-and-go hair. That was fantastic!

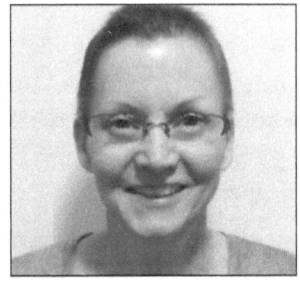

Wash-and-go hair.
Photo by Mark Ormsby.

* * *

Later that same evening, there was another surprise. Only, that one was not so good.

My first round of chemo and white blood cell injection were catching up with me. I was sprawled out on our living room couch feeling exhausted. My teens were doing homework in their rooms, and my husband was working quietly in a nearby room so I could have some peace and quiet. I fell into a deep sleep.

"Bam! Bam! Bam!"

"Bam! Bam! Bam!"

"Get outta here!" "Get outta here!" "Get outta here!" Mark yelled.

What on Earth was going on?

Was this a dream?

I was shaking from being so startled. Apparently, this was not a dream.

Our dog, Colby, was barking. Mark is usually a calm, quiet man. I knew emotions were high in our home at that time, but I could not imagine what had made him so upset.

Still feeling groggy, I sat up on the couch to see what was happening.

Colby was standing in our foyer barking at the closed front doors of our home. Mark was nearby in our family room waiting for the strangers to leave. He did not want to open the door again.

I looked outside our front picture window and saw two people, a man and a woman, standing on our front porch. The man was five feet from the door. The woman was closer.

I was finally alert enough to realize that Mark was yelling at them because they were selling something at our door, and they were not even wearing masks! And my immune system was weaker than it had been two days prior.

A few minutes later they drove away.

There was a pandemic out there.

Did they not get the memo?

* * *

It was an interesting three-week cycle between my first and second rounds of chemo. As I previously mentioned, I did some research on chemo side effects. I knew there could be some stomach issues. However, other problems occurred that I had not expected.

Not knowing how chemo might affect me personally, I was physically prepared for anything. I had two different medications Dr. N prescribed for nausea and various over-the-counter medicines already in the house. And the thoughtful package my sister-in-law sent ahead of time included wristbands that used acupressure to help with chemotherapy-induced nausea.

For the first few days following chemo, I took the first prescription from Dr. N. I also wore the wristbands for about a week after my first round. Those were more as a precaution.

I didn't feel nauseous at all. It's hard to say which precaution worked best for me, so I was glad I used both. I was also glad to have had options for over-the-counter medicines for my stomach since I had some discomfort.

As far as other side effects were concerned, I was quite tired for a few days after my treatment. I read that the fatigue

I was feeling was because my body was working extra hard to repair the damage from the chemo treatment. Fortunately, it was also getting rid of the cancer.

I've always been an active person. I can relax but not for long. I feel better about myself when I'm being "productive." So, during that three-week cycle, I had to force myself to rest at times during the day.

I realized that resting, when I needed it after chemo, was a way to be productive. It helped me "refuel" from time to time to keep my energy level up throughout the day.

* * *

Five nights after my first round of chemo I woke up with an unusual pain. Trying hard not to panic, I nudged my husband.

"My back!"

"What's wrong?" asked Mark.

"I'm getting shooting pains down my back! I've never had that before!"

"All of a sudden? What do you think it's from?"

"I have no idea!"

"Your chemo treatment was almost a week ago. It doesn't seem like that would suddenly start causing you pain now, does it?"

"No, it doesn't."

I did my best to sleep despite the sharp pains going up and down my back. I was hoping it would be better by morning.

The next morning, I got up from my bed. Then I sat back down.

"My back still hurts," I told Mark.

"What exactly makes it hurt?"

"It hurts when I stand up, bend over to sit, or lie on my back. It feels like a painful rollercoaster going up and down my spine."

"Let's contact your doctor," he suggested.

"I can't believe this is happening. Why do I have so much trouble with medicines?"

I sent a message to Dr. N through the patient portal.

Once they gave me Benadryl the chemo meds were okay. Since then, I've had some troubles with my stomach but have been able to somewhat keep that under control. My temperature went up to 100.4 yesterday afternoon. I called the hospital. They said I had to come in if it went up to 100.5 because of COVID. It didn't go any higher and I've been fever free since yesterday evening. For some reason, I woke up last night with horrible back spasms.

The waves of pain in my back continued for three days.

Dr. N suggested I tell my primary care doctor about the reaction. My doctor gave me some home back exercises and suggested I take an over-the-counter pain medicine. I wasn't sure if the exercises or other medicine helped, but the pain subsided after a while.

* * *

As I approached the end of the three-week cycle, I found more and more strands of my hair on the bathroom sink. It was starting to go. So glad my hair was short already.

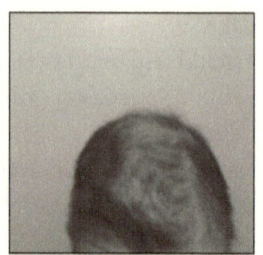

Going...Going. *Photo by Mark Ormsby*

* * *

A couple of days later, I was back at the hospital for round two. As I was walking up to the table in the front lobby, I saw a woman facing her phone toward the guard sitting there. Then I heard the guard say something to her.

"Looks like you're cleared for COVID-19."

All I needed to do was show the guard the answered questions on my phone. I didn't have to keep answering the same questions three times for my appointments. Great! Feeling smarter than I did when I left my house that morning, I approached the guard with my phone and showed him my green COVID screen.

"Great! You're good to go!"

Wow. That made so much more sense than last time. All I had to do was keep showing people I had already answered the questions and I was set.

My next stop was the oncology department. That time when I entered there was nobody waiting in line. So, I walked up to the sticker on the floor closest to the desk. I turned my phone around to show her I had already answered the COVID questions.

"Have you recently traveled to New York?" she asked.

"No, I haven't." I kept my phone facing her so she'd notice once she looked up at me.

"Have you been in close contact with anyone who tested positive for COVID-19 in the last fourteen days?"

"No, I haven't, but—"

"Do you currently have a fever or chills, cough, shortness of breath, fatigue, nausea or vomiting, diarrhea, or muscle or body aches?" she continued.

"No, but—"

"I see you showing me you answered the COVID-19 questions. We still need to ask here at this check-in anyway."

Bummer. Just when I thought I had it figured out, wrong again. I also thought it would make her day if she didn't have to ask every single person going in there the same questions. Oh well.

* * *

Naturally, I was quite nervous about the second round. The thought of another bad reaction consumed me. I wondered if my nurse for this round was up to speed on my treatments.

I decided to talk to her about my chemo. For some reason, the nurse who was assigned to me that day left early on and never came back. A different nurse came in to tell me she was filling in for her.

"I'll get you started since your nurse isn't available right now."

"Okay. Thanks. Since I reacted badly to the first treatment, will I be given Benadryl again?"

She skimmed through my online chart. "Yes. I'll give you 25 milligrams of Benadryl before you get the first chemo medicine."

I didn't want to tell her how to do her job. Still, I was nervous about having another bad reaction. It was hard to tell how many patients she saw throughout the day. It seemed like it would be hard to keep track of everyone's treatment details.

I trusted she looked closely enough at my chart and would completely prepare me for the chemo medicine. That round needed to be shorter since I had to be home in time for my senior's virtual high school graduation.

"Okay. So, I just gave you the Benadryl," she said. "I'll be back soon to start your first chemo med."

About twenty minutes later that same nurse came back and hooked another bag to the pole.

"There," she said. "I started your first chemo medicine."

I waited nervously as she left my room. Maybe two minutes later, I called her back. I could not believe I was having the same bad reaction! I knew she gave me Benadryl. I couldn't figure out why that was happening again. Once again, Nurse J came in to help.

"You're having another bad reaction to your med," said Nurse J.

"Did you give her Benadryl before the chemo medicine?" she asked my nurse.

"Yes, I gave her 25 milligrams like she had last time. But I'm not her nurse today."

"We'll give you another 25 milligrams and see if that calms things down," Nurse J said.

The extra 25 milligrams helped. I didn't understand. Why was I still reacting? Now I need twice as much Benadryl? What was going to happen during the third and fourth rounds of chemo? Would they have to keep adding more Benadryl each time?

A nurse practitioner on staff came in to help figure out why I was still reacting badly.

"You gave her the Benadryl before the first chemo med?"

"Yes, I did," my nurse said.

Her eyes slowly moved through my online chart. "Did you also start her on a slow drip?"

"Um…I don't think so."

"She needs to be on a slow drip. It's in her chart."

"Well, she's not really my patient. I'm filling in for someone."

It was all I could do to keep my mouth shut. For once, I was relieved to have a mask covering my face. I know she's only human, and maybe she was doing a lot, but I was angry that she wasn't looking closer at my chart. I trusted her and was afraid she might be insulted if I had told her about the slow drip too. I gave her the benefit of the doubt.

Although there were some side effects of the Benadryl again, at least it helped me get through the chemo treatment once again.

Since they switched to a slow drip the treatment took longer than planned again. A few more hours passed. I wondered if I would make it home in time for the graduation. I was tired and my legs were feeling restless. I just wanted to go home.

I kept updating Mark through text messages. Since the hospital was about thirty minutes from home, I was trying to time it so he would get there as soon as I was done. Of course, neither of us wanted to miss the event.

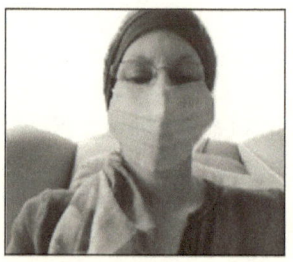

Wanting to go home.
Photo by Wendy Ormsby.

We made it home with only a few minutes to spare! Although the school did a great job of showing senior pictures of the graduates, with details of each student's future, it wasn't the same as a live graduation.

It was heartbreaking watching our graduate sit in front of the television on graduation day instead of walking across a stage. However, it did mean that I could "attend" the ceremony.

* * *

I returned to the hospital the next morning for my second white blood cell injection. As far as giving myself the injection, once I saw the notes on how to do it, I opted to take my chances and have a nurse do it at the hospital. Fortunately, everything went smoothly.

Four days after my white blood cell injection, the back spasms started up again. There was no way to know for sure what the cause was the first time. After talking to Dr. N about my second round of chemo and the returning spasms, she concluded that the spasms were from the injection.

"That's not a likely reaction to that injection. But it makes even less sense that it would be from the chemo meds. So, it must be the injection," she confirmed.

"I still need it though, don't I?"

"Yes. I'm afraid so, especially during a pandemic."

"At least I only need it two more times."

My feelings did not match my optimistic words.

"Yes. And, as far as your chemo treatments are concerned, I'm going to have them give you more medicine before they give you the chemo meds. You'll be getting two steroids to help prevent a bad reaction to the first chemo med. I didn't want to give you those initially since you have diabetes, and they can raise your blood sugar. I think that's what we'll have to do, though. I'll also speak to your endocrinologist to make sure she knows, and she can prescribe something to bring your blood glucose down if it gets too high."

I loved that Dr. N was communicating so well with my endocrinologist! I also had my fingers crossed, said a little prayer, and hoped for the best during my last two appointments.

* * *

I had an appointment with Dr. N minutes before my third round. She had a way of keeping my hopes up even when I encountered setbacks.

"Hello. You're halfway there," Dr. N said with a smile.

"Yes, I am. May I ask you something?"

"Sure."

"I'm glad I'll have more meds to hopefully prevent a bad reaction this time. Is there a way you can make sure that my nurse will use a slow drip for my first chemo med, please?"

"Yes. I'll make sure it's in your chart."

I was feeling quite apprehensive. It would've been nice if the confidence I had in my future nurses matched the confidence I had in my doctor. Plus, I didn't know who my nurse would be each time.

Dr. N and I were done talking and, as I was sitting there in the small infusion center room waiting for my nurse, I decided to turn on the television. Since I could be there for hours, I thought a distraction might be good. I didn't want to disturb the other patients, so I turned the volume down low and used the captions.

My nurse for that round entered my room. Oh boy. It was the same one who substituted during my last round of chemo. Only now she would have to add more medicine to my regimen. I could no longer give her the benefit of the doubt.

"Are you giving me two steroids before the Benadryl?" I asked her.

Her eyes glanced at my online chart. "Yes. It looks like you need two steroids, then 50 milligrams of Benadryl, before you get your chemo meds."

"Okay. And are you going to set the first chemo med to a slow drip?"

She glimpsed at my chart again. "Only the first chemo med will have a slow drip."

"Right, that's the one I'm allergic to so…"

I was no longer worried about insulting her. If she wasn't going to take the time to completely understand my treatment plan, then I was going to make sure it was done right. Maybe I sounded like a know-it-all, but I didn't care. It was my health and possibly my life at stake. The saline had been going for a while, so she started the first steroid and then the second one.

Eventually, she started the 50 milligrams of Benadryl. Once again, I was sleepy and then jittery. Apparently, it was the Benadryl that made me feel that way last time. Great. Guess it was the lesser of two evils since I still needed it to get through the chemotherapy treatments.

"Okay. Time for your first chemo med."

"I'm nervous."

"Don't worry. You'll be fine. When it's done just use the call button. It's hard to tell from the hallway which room has the machine that's going off when the medicine is done," she said.

Soon after the chemo medicine started an alarm went off on the machine. I pushed the call button. My nurse came back to the room.

"Hm. I don't know why it's going off like that," she said.

"I don't know either." I stared at her in disbelief.

She stopped the alarm and started the chemo medicine again. Maybe twenty minutes later, the alarm went off again. That time I looked closely at the machine. It said something about air being in the tube. So, I pushed the call button again. Soon after, she was back in my room.

"What is going on with your machine today? This doesn't usually happen."

"I noticed there's a message that says, 'air in tube' when the alarm is going off like that," I said.

"It's probably nothing."

Probably nothing? The real question was what was going on with that nurse? The alarm went off several more times throughout the treatment. Talk about stress! I promise I was not touching anything on the machine. I finally made it through both chemo medicines. Whew!

* * *

The next day I had my third white blood cell injection. The hospital seemed empty. It was the day before a major holiday, and many employees went home early. Amid cancer treatments and a pandemic, it was easy for holidays and other important events to get lost in the shuffle.

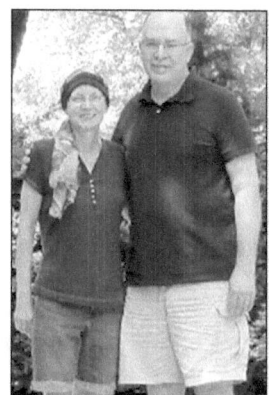

It was also our twenty-first wedding anniversary. Our family was still able to go to the grove where Mark and I were married. It had been our tradition to take annual pictures there to celebrate the day. I knew I wasn't looking my best. We carried on our tradition anyway.

Happy anniversary.
Photo by Ezra Ormsby

* * *

Along with the usual back spasms four days after the injection, I ended up feeling more nauseous after the third round of chemo. That was strange. Luckily, it didn't last long, though. And the spasms only lasted two days instead of four this time. I was so glad to have three rounds down and only one more to go.

* * *

It was about halfway between my third and fourth rounds of chemo when my parents called me. There was a family wedding about to take place in the Midwest, so I figured they were calling me about that. Not exactly.

"I'm calling to tell you that I have skin cancer," said my dad.

"Skin cancer? Do you happen to know what kind?"

"Squamous cell carcinoma. My doctor said I won't need chemo, though."

While we were talking, I typed "squamous cell carcinoma" on my computer. I read some details to him out loud.

He was impressed that I knew so much about it. I really didn't. By that time, I had learned where to find reliable information on cancer quickly. I had been using the Mayo Clinic site for months.

"My surgery is scheduled for next week. That's why we aren't going to the wedding. My doctor said I can't go anywhere, especially with a pandemic going on."

"Makes sense to me," I said.

I called my dad the day after his surgery. Thankfully, it was a success. He reassured me that he was going to be okay. It was one less thing to worry about.

* * *

Before I continued my chemo treatments, I was due for another bilateral mammogram. It seemed odd, after everything I had already done, that I still needed one. Fortunately, nothing suspicious was found.

* * *

Still wearing a mask, I went to the hospital for my last round of chemo. I made it past the front door security and the front desk in the oncology unit without any problems.

I had thank you cards for the staff in the oncology unit. One was for the women at the front desk. Another was for the nursing staff. I'm sure that can be a thankless job at times.

My nurse for the last round of chemo was amazing. They saved the best for last! Nurse A was attentive and seemed quite confident in what she was doing the entire time. I knew from the start that it was going to be a great way to finish my chemo treatments.

"Good morning, Ms. Ormsby. How are you feeling today?"

"Good morning. I'm okay, I guess. Just nervous since I've had so many problems."

"I'm going to make sure everything is done very carefully so you don't have any more problems."

Nurse A gave me the saline, then the two steroids, then the Benadryl. She continued to check on me while I was receiving the medicines. She came back to the room again to start the first chemo medicine and offered to stay in the room with me.

"I can stay in here for as long as you like," she said.

"Really? Yes, please!"

"Not a problem. I can do my work right here on this computer."

"By the way, I have something for you and the other nurses." I handed the thank you card to Nurse A. She was pleasantly surprised.

Since she checked on me so often, and I didn't have any problems, this was the shortest round. As soon as one medicine was done, she was there to start the next one. The best part of that appointment was the last thing Nurse A did for me.

"Congratulations! You finished your chemo!" She sang as she danced back into my room. "Here is your certificate."

"My certificate?"

"That's right. It's a certificate of achievement for finishing chemo treatments and some of the nurses signed it."

As I was leaving the oncology unit, Nurse A escorted me over to a counter and told me to ring the bell that was sitting on it.

I hesitated at first because I wasn't sure I wanted to draw that much attention to myself. Then I thought, what the heck! As I was ringing the bell it was as if people were coming out of the woodwork! Everyone was clapping for me! That felt great.

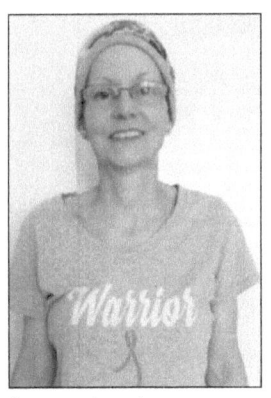

Although I wasn't physically up to celebrating the end of chemo, my husband and two older teens fixed a delicious dinner for us that evening. They also made sure I was able to relax for the rest of the evening and

No more chemo!
Photo by Mark Ormsby

the next few days. I was so happy to be done with chemo and grateful for their support throughout my treatments.

❋ ❋ ❋

I was back the next day for my final injection. To my surprise, Nurse A was there! She was not the nurse who was scheduled to give me the injection. However, when she saw me waiting for a while, she let me know that if my nurse didn't show up soon, she would do it for me. Like I said, what an amazing person!

Although I continued to have mild chemo side effects, I knew I did not have COVID. My breathing was fine throughout my treatments. I did not have a sore throat, and I was not congested or coughing. It became easier to recognize the differences between COVID symptoms and chemo side effects. Next, I had to prepare for radiation treatments both mentally and physically.

- 6 -

Pain Endured

CHEMO ENDED AND I WAS SCHEDULED FOR A COVID-19 TEST. It wasn't because I had any symptoms or thought I had been exposed to it. It was a requirement before I could receive radiation treatments. Odd that I didn't need that before I started chemo.

It took a few days, but my COVID test results were back. Still negative. Whew! I was back at the radiation center for my simulation. That was interesting.

At our meeting months before, Dr. F did a great job of describing what would take place at the simulation and during treatments. Still, some steps seemed easier to understand once they were happening.

Before I started the simulation, Nurse M, whom I had already met, gave me a tour of the center. She showed me what to do when I arrived for my daily treatments. She also gave me a card to scan at the front desk every day so I could get started as soon as possible.

To start the simulation, I was escorted into a small brightly lit room that had a CT scanner in the middle of it. The table that the scanner encircled had a large flexible pad at the head of it.

First, the radiation therapist needed to find the best position for my body to give me the best treatment. She told me to lie down so she could create a mold for my head, shoulders, and arms using the large flexible pad.

Once the mold was made, it was supposed to keep that shape and help me stay in that same position for every treatment. That way, the beams hit the same target area every time. Genius idea!

As I was lying face up, with my forearms and hands resting above my head, I could feel my shoulder blades digging into the flexible but firm pad. I started feeling mild shooting pains up and down my left arm.

"How long will I have to be in this position?" I asked the therapist.

"It shouldn't take more than twenty minutes to measure," she said. "I'm going to use a marker to draw on you because it will help us align your body to the laser lights every time."

She drew Xs on round quarter-sized translucent stickers already on several areas of my upper torso. "You must keep these stickers on throughout your treatments, so they know where to aim the radiation. I'm also going to give you small tattoos on both sides of your torso, and one in the middle of your chest, to mark where the beams will be."

"So, I can't wash off the marks until all my radiation treatments are done?"

"If they accidentally come off, don't worry, we'll just measure again."

"Okay. And are the tattoos permanent?" I asked. "Yes. Don't worry though. They're so small you won't even notice them. They're about the size of the tip of a ballpoint pen."

She was friendly but the last thing I wanted was to go through this simulation again. I wasn't sure how I was going to keep the marks on my skin for a month. Even so, I was determined to do it somehow.

She was also kind enough to let me bring my arms down between the different steps of the simulation. That helped keep the pain in my arm to a minimum.

She told me the next step involved holding my breath. Throughout that appointment, my mask had been covering my nose and mouth. She left the room for a moment then came back with a machine with a flexible tube attached to it.

"Have you ever gone snorkeling before?"

"No. I'm not much of a swimmer, actually," I admitted. "Oh. Well, I'll need you to take your mask off and put the mouthpiece on this tube in your mouth. I'm going to give you nose plugs, too. We need to see how long you can hold your breath. Once we know you can hold your breath long enough, I can take some CT scans of your treatment area. Holding your breath during the scanning decreases movement inside your body. That way we can get the clearest images for your treatment plan," she explained.

"I'll try but I've never been very good at holding my breath underwater when I swim."

"We'll start with holding for five seconds then work our way up to thirty-five seconds." She tried hard to encourage me. I really appreciated it.

"Thirty-five seconds? That seems like a long time to hold my breath."

"You can do this. I'm not a good swimmer either. In fact, I never swim underwater. So, you're way ahead of me."

I practiced holding my breath with the machine over and over until I could hold it for thirty-five seconds. The therapist left the room and returned with someone else to confirm that I could hold my breath long enough for the CT scan. I couldn't believe I could hold it for that long.

"She can hold her breath for thirty-five seconds," she told him.

"Great!" He looked at me and said, "Can you hold it for *forty* seconds?"

"Uh, I'll try. I mean, what's another five seconds, right?"

I was really hoping I could make it to forty seconds. If not, I wasn't sure what I would have to do. Of course, I wanted the images from the scan as clear as possible. Like the therapist said, clearer images would be helpful for the treatment plan. Luckily, I could hold my breath for forty seconds. Then I was ready for the CT scan.

Being as claustrophobic as I am, it was good that I already had a CT scan months before that appointment. In other words, I already knew that it wouldn't feel nearly as claustrophobic as an MRI machine. It looked like a big donut instead of a tunnel.

That part of my simulation did not take long at all. I went through the machine a few times holding my breath each time to get the images. And the entire simulation was done.

* * *

About four weeks later, I started the radiation treatments. Like I was taught on the day of my simulation, I entered the radiation center, showed the receptionist the note on my phone showing I was negative for COVID-19 symptoms, then scanned my entry card at the front desk. I was good to go. Or so I thought.

I sat with a cloth gown on from the waist up in a small waiting area reserved for women only. Across the narrow hall was another waiting area for both women and men. I was grateful that they offered space for only women to sit together. Of course, we still had to sit six feet apart. On the wall of that small waiting area were two signs. The pandemic was still going strong. The messages on those signs made me feel heavy-hearted for a moment.

One sign read, "HELP KEEP OUR HOSPITAL AND COMMUNITY SAFE. NO VISITORS ARE ALLOWED."

The other one stated, "PLEASE PRACTICE SOCIAL DISTANCING HERE. Maintain 6 feet of distance from others, avoid crowded public places where close contact with others may occur, avoid mass gatherings."

I was glad they put those signs in there. However, it was heartbreaking to be reminded of the pandemic so clearly while I was there alone getting more cancer treatments.

At least I didn't have to wait long before I was called back. I was politely greeted by a radiation therapist wearing a mask. After he introduced himself, Therapist P asked me a few questions: "What is your name and date of birth?" "Have you recently tested positive for COVID-19?" "Have you recently been around anyone who tested positive for COVID-19?" "Have you recently been to a nursing facility?"

That was about the extent of his questions. After all, I did answer those and several other COVID-19 questions before I arrived for my appointment. Those same questions were asked every time I went to the back to start my radiation treatments.

I was glad they were being so vigilant there. After the questions, he asked me to put my hands out and proceeded to spray foam hand sanitizer on them. Like I said, vigilant!

I followed Therapist P into a large room that had a high and rather unique ceiling. There was a two-dimensional palm tree drawing and other relaxing images. Across the room was a table with a machine hanging over it.

The mold they made during my simulation was at the head of the table. Therapist P asked me to put my bag on a nearby chair and then lie down on the table. So far so good.

One part of the machine was maybe two feet above me, aimed at my chest. A tech helping Therapist P opened my gown and turned on the laser lights. Fortunately, the marker did not wash off during the many showers I had since the simulation day.

Therapist P put more stickers on me and drew more Xs with a marker. They really were precise with those treatments.

"We have to do a 'dry run' by taking images before we can start your treatment," he said.

"Are you only doing that today?" I tried to smile.

"We'll be doing that once a week. So, plan on staying longer on those days. We'll also have to take measurements each time. It should take a lot less time after the first couple of days."

Although I appreciated how precisely they wanted to deliver the radiation each time, I didn't understand why the images and measurements were taking so long. I knew it was the first day of radiation, but I was lying there for at least twenty-five minutes. My arms were above my head like in the simulation. However, I had to keep my arms above my head a lot longer.

Sometimes, taking deep breaths through painful moments can help ease the pain. The problem was, I was wearing a mask. That made deep breathing difficult. As the pain in my left shoulder and arm were increasing, I knew I needed to say something.

"Can I put my arms down briefly?"

"I'm sorry. If you move, then we'll have to start over. Moving even your arms will change your position too much," said Therapist P.

"I'm feeling a lot of pain in my left shoulder and arm."

"Sorry about your pain. We'll work as fast as we can so you can bring your arms down."

The longer I stayed on that table with my arms over my head, the more intense the pain grew. Eventually, it traveled from my shoulder all the way down my left arm and into my hand. It was all throbbing.

Two thoughts helped me get through that first day of radiation. One was that it was hopefully helping me get rid of any remaining cancer cells. And the other was what Therapist P said. I trusted that he understood my pain and was working as fast as he could.

The next day was even more of a challenge. After going through the check-in routine, changing into a gown, and waiting for my turn, a therapist escorted me to the same room for my treatment. There, across the room, was that table again. And on that table was that mold.

"Okay. We're going to take some images and measurements again."

"I thought the images were only once a week." I didn't mean to be a pain, but I wasn't sure I could bear being in that position for a long time again.

"We need to take more for today's treatment. After today, it shouldn't take as long to set things up."

I was worried that if it took as long as it did the day before then I would have that immense pain in my left shoulder and arm again. Sure enough, that time on the table also took about twenty-five minutes. And that tremendous pain returned. It was all I could do not to cry.

Then, about five minutes before it was done, I couldn't take it anymore. Tears started rolling down my face and into my mask. Crying with a mask on was not a good feeling. Still, I was hoping that meant nobody knew I was crying. For some reason, I was trying to be stoic.

I left the second day of radiation feeling exhausted. On the third day, I decided to ask Therapist P a question before I was even at the table.

"Are we going to do more images and measurements today?"

"Yes, but it shouldn't take as long as the first two days."

"I don't think I can do this again. If I need to lie here with my arms over my head for a while, then I'd rather not do this at all."

I knew I needed radiation. I trusted Dr. F and Dr. N. However, I couldn't see myself lying there again in that painful position. I knew something had to change. Seeing how upset I was, Therapist P suggested something.

"How about if you talk to your doctor before we do this again?"

"I can do that. When?"

"Do you have time to wait this morning? I'll see if she has a few minutes between scheduled patients to talk to you."

"Really?"

"Yes. Are you okay waiting in the bigger waiting room?" he asked.

"Sure, I can do that. Thank you so much for understanding."

"You're welcome. Hope we can come up with an easier way for you to get through your treatments."

"I hope so too."

* * *

After a short wait, I talked to Dr. F. To my surprise, she asked if I could stay so they could make a new mold. The goal was to make one that didn't put such a strain on my left shoulder.

Unfortunately, I still needed to keep my arms over my head while I was on the table.

I tried to mentally prepare myself to go through all the measuring, breathing, and CT scans again. I had a different therapist that time. Everyone at that place was so polite.

The therapist started by putting a new pad down to make a different mold for me. He took more measurements and put more stickers and Xs on me. That didn't take long at all. There wasn't a big difference in the way my arms were placed over my head, but it was a little more comfortable. I returned to the radiation center five days later to start over again. Luckily, the shoulder pain was no longer an issue.

* * *

I spent my first three appointments alone in the waiting room. Maybe they weren't as busy because of the pandemic. I didn't have to wait long each time. Of course, it was still easy to think about things a lot. I was really hoping everything would run smoothly for the rest of my radiation treatments.

* * *

As I entered the waiting room area on the first day starting my treatments over, I was surprised to see another woman in the smaller "women only" waiting room. With a mask on her face, it was hard to tell how friendly she might be. I noticed she was wearing a beautiful silk scarf on her head since she had also lost her hair from chemo.

Even if she wasn't that sociable, I was still happy to see another female patient in here. I don't have a naturally loud voice. I was hoping that if I said hello through my mask, she'd hear me.

"Good morning," I said.

"Good morning," she replied.

Okay. Good. She could hear me through my mask. Now

what? Talking to another cancer patient while waiting for an appointment can be difficult. What do you say to a total stranger who is there for a similar worrisome reason as you?

"This pandemic is just crazy, huh?"

Probably wasn't the best thing to say.

"Yes, it is."

"I didn't see you here last week. Is this your first week of radiation?" I asked.

"I started last week but this will be my regular time for appointments. How about you?"

"It's kind of a long story. I initially started on August 11th. Then, after two days of not being able to comfortably lie in that position, they decided to make a new mold for me. Now, I'm starting over this week. So, technically, this is my first of four weeks."

"I see. Sorry you had to start over again."

She seemed friendly and sophisticated. I enjoyed talking with her. It was comforting having someone else there, especially since my husband couldn't be there with me. We continued talking until I was called back for my turn.

＊ ＊ ＊

The next day that same woman was in the waiting room when I arrived. That time I thought to ask her name.

"Hello again." I sat down leaving a few seats between us.

"Oh hi."

"My name is Wendy, by the way."

"I'm Jill."

"Nice to officially meet you, Jill."

"Nice to meet you too," she said with a smile.

"You know, Jill, I have this gray scarf here that I ordered online. Turns out it doesn't fit me. It seems that I have the world's smallest head," I laughed. "Would you like the scarf? I'm guessing it will look a lot better on you."

"Sure. I'll try it. Thanks so much."

A therapist called me back for my turn in the radiation room. Even though Jill was there before me on both days, her appointments seemed to be after mine. Now that we had officially met, I tried to arrive a little early every day so we would have more time to talk. It was lonely getting cancer treatments during a pandemic.

* * *

The next day Jill was there when I arrived. This time, she was wearing something familiar to me.

"That scarf looks great on you!" I said.

"Thanks. And thanks for the scarf."

"You're welcome. I'm glad I have someone to give it to, and it fits you so much better than me."

The time we had wasn't long. However, it was still nice.

Later the same week, I told Jill about my oldest child heading off to college for the first time. She wished me good luck with everything.

* * *

It was time to take my oldest to college. It was bizarre to think that life was still going on during my cancer treatments and the pandemic. I mean, of course, it was. And, as it turned out, taking my child to college was a great distraction.

Because of the pandemic, the school was at one-third capacity for students. My child had a suitemate, and, when we arrived on move-in day, the suitemate and her family were also there. The two of them had previously met through Zoom, and the suitemate knew about my cancer.

As I was standing there with my husband and our college-bound student in the dorm room, the suitemate and her family cut through the shared bathroom to meet us. Her family of five were all there, and they were all wearing masks and keeping a safe distance from us.

Of course, I was happy to meet the family. However, I knew I didn't look my best. My hair had thinned out a lot, so I was wearing a chemo cap. I had also lost a little more weight during the chemo treatments, so I was looking quite thin. Then I remembered something crucial. I was still alive. Because of that, I could see my oldest child off to college.

Despite how I may have looked, none of them seemed uncomfortable around me. I was grateful for that. The suitemates hit it off, and the move-in day was a big success all around! The day after move-in day, the second week of my revised radiation treatments began.

* * *

At the start of the second week, I met another friendly woman. She finished her appointment and stopped by the waiting room to talk to Jill. They seemed to be finishing a conversation they started before she was called back for her turn. She saw me sitting there and Jill introduced us.

"Wendy, this is Donna."

"Hi, Donna," I replied.

"Well, now I'm off to chemo!" Donna said.

What? She was leaving her radiation appointment and going straight to a chemo treatment? Well, if I was going to see so few other patients, these two would be the best ones to see.

Since Donna was on her way out, we didn't say anything else to each other. There was no sign of Donna for the rest of the week. I wondered what that was about.

Donna's cancer was different from mine and Jill's. It was in her mouth and throat. I could only imagine how terrifying that would be.

If I hadn't met Donna at a cancer treatment center, I probably wouldn't have even known she had cancer. She looked quite healthy and had a bubbly personality. It felt good being around that positive energy with everything that was going on.

* * *

As the treatments continued, Jill and I had deeper conversations. And, from that, I could tell a true friendship was forming. She told me a few things about her breast cancer, including having it for a second time, and the fact that her husband had died in 2019. She wasn't there every day because of a slight shift in her schedule. It didn't feel the same without her.

Even though I was not seeing Donna nearly as much, I could tell we were all becoming good friends and wanted to stay in touch. These new friendships were something to look forward to after active cancer treatments were done.

A peculiar coincidence occurred at the radiation center

that convinced us, even more, to keep in touch. I must have left my house extra early that day because both Donna and Jill were in the waiting room when I arrived. The therapist called Donna back, and I could hear her when he asked for her birthdate.

"9/17…"

That was all I could hear. Donna finished before I was called back and stopped by the waiting room to say goodbye.

"Hey, Donna, did I hear you say your birthday is '9/17'?"

"Yes!"

"Mine too!"

"Really?! That's great! And our birthday is coming up soon!" she pointed out.

* * *

The following Monday Jill was there and surprised me with a message from Donna.

"Donna wants to take us out to lunch for your birthdays."

"I would love to do that!"

Of course, we were still in the thick of a pandemic. My own family hadn't eaten at any restaurants for months. I wasn't sure how that would even work. I was interested in joining them if we could find a safe way to do it. After all, we were all immunocompromised.

Jill and I also talked about our medical oncologists. As she started talking about her doctor, something dawned on me. She had one of the same doctors I had before I found Dr. N. Oh boy. I don't like receiving unsolicited advice, so I try my best not to give it. I figured this time I had to make an exception.

At first, I stayed quiet about it. However, the more Jill talked about this doctor the more I wanted to say something. She appreciated the support. Apparently, she was already looking into finding a different medical oncologist anyway.

* * *

I was about halfway through my month of radiation treatments when something happened on my way out of an appointment. I always parked in the same garage in front of the building. It was one of the longer days where they needed to take more measurements. I was so glad to be done for the day.

After I pulled out of my space with my minivan, I noticed a woman driving a compact car was having trouble leaving the garage. She didn't notice that the gate was already up in front of her. Since I was pulling out from a side aisle, my van was perpendicular to her car and at least a car length away.

As she kept trying to put her ticket in the machine, another woman pulled up behind her, leaving enough space for me to turn right and then forward to the machine once that first woman was through. I wondered why she didn't see that the gate was up for her. The next thing I knew, the woman at the gate was backing up!

What was even more puzzling, as she was backing up, she turned toward me for some odd reason. Once I realized that I laid on my horn. When I say I "laid" on it I mean I pushed it as hard as I could for what seemed like ten seconds. It didn't matter though.

"Bam!" Her car smashed into the front of my van.

After that, she moved forward again, still determined to

get out of the garage. Considering she hit my van, she was not going anywhere just yet. I stepped out of my van and walked over to her driver's side window. Only after I started talking to her, I noticed I was not wearing my mask. My mind was on other things that day.

"You just hit my van!" I said loudly while pointing to my van behind her. My hands and voice were quivering.

She tried to explain that she could not get out of the garage, ignoring the fact that she shouldn't leave anyway because she hit my vehicle. Since she still hadn't noticed the gate was up, I no longer worried about her leaving.

"You just hit my van!" I repeated. "You can't leave until we exchange information."

"Let's pull over here," she said as she pointed to a spot away from the gate.

At least the other woman not involved could finally get out of there. I also loved the fact that she was telling me where to park my van. We pulled over away from the gate and stepped out of our vehicles to assess the damage. It was quite noticeable on my van. We exchanged information, then I headed home. I was already in a bad mood. That did not help.

It was a real chore getting her insurance company to pay for the damage. That was the last thing I wanted to deal with during those months of treatments. One good thing was that nobody was hurt. As for her gate confusion, may God help her in the future.

✹ ✹ ✹

It was the weekend before my last two radiation treatments.

Cedar Ridge was holding an outdoor service after months of having them on Zoom. They wanted to try face-to-face before the weather turned too cold. There was plenty of space to sit far enough away from each other and still participate in the service.

Since this was late in the year, and had been a very challenging year for many, our Lead Pastor, Matthew, asked if anyone wanted to share their ups and downs of the year 2020. I have never been comfortable with public speaking. However, this is a church where everyone feels welcome, and nobody judges. If anyone could get anything out of my experiences, then why not share them?

One person walked up to the microphone. He mentioned how he was glad we were able to have the Zoom services.

I hesitated to go up there.

Since I didn't see anyone else walking up at that moment, I made my way to the front. As Pastor Matthew was cleaning off the microphone with an alcohol wipe, I thought about what to say. I took off my mask and started speaking.

"Hello, everyone. My name is Wendy and some of you already know that I was diagnosed with invasive breast cancer earlier this year." My voice was trembling. "I've had a lot of setbacks this year concerning my cancer treatments. I've also had a lot of compassion, support, prayers, and great doctors to help me get through it all. Thank you to everyone who's been there for me." I smiled at Pastor Ruth who was standing off to the side. "Now I'm almost done with treatments, and I will survive 2020! Thanks again!"

* * *

The weekend was over, and I finished my last two days of radiation treatments. I was sore, exhausted, and looked like a cooked lobster. Still, I was done! I made it! As I did on my last day of chemo, I gave thank you cards to the staff.

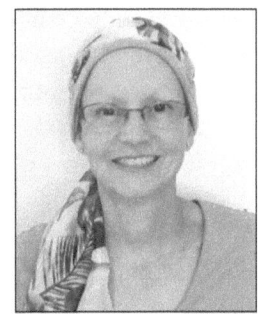

Radiation is done!
Photo by Mark Ormsby.

The first card was handed to Therapist P. It was addressed to the entire team, but he was the one who helped me the most. The second was for Dr. F. She listened when I mentioned needing a medical oncologist, and she showed compassion throughout my radiation treatments.

Last, but not least, was the card for Nurse M. I knew I would be seeing at least Nurse M and Dr. F again, but I wanted to thank them that day anyway.

"Oh, my goodness, thank you!" said Nurse M. "That is so nice of you." She read the card and then crossed her arms over her chest to simulate a hug.

It's moments like that when a pandemic can take away sincere gratitude. However, Nurse M was very clear about her appreciation for thanking her. She really did make my time at the radiation center much more bearable. Plus, she was the one who directed me toward my physical therapist who was so helpful.

"And now, I have something for you," said Nurse M.

She had a folder in her hand and pulled out a diploma with my name on it. It also had the names of a lot of staff members at the radiation center. It was a sure sign that I had successfully completed my radiation treatments!

I walked out of the center that day relieved that the treatments were over and I was able to finish them after all. Another step toward recovery was done! And, as a special bonus, I made two amazing friends in the process!

Two days later Jill, Donna, and I met at a restaurant with outdoor seating. They were both there already when I arrived. It was strange seeing them without masks. Jill didn't have a scarf on either. I almost didn't recognize either of them! We exchanged birthday gifts and enjoyed our lunch together. The three of us decided to stay in touch after our birthday celebration.

※ ※ ※

Dr. N wanted me to come in for a follow-up appointment. She said it was okay to wait until my skin healed enough from radiation treatments first.

- 7 -

No Evidence

Before I went to my follow-up with Dr. N, I heard the news of my dear friend Colleen Heitkamp passing away on September 24, 2020. I will always be grateful for her tremendous support and insight and her profound words and kindness even when she was not at her best.

* * *

A couple of weeks after my radiation treatments were done, I saw Dr. N again. I already had some questions for her about my immune system, vaccines, and the medicine she would be prescribing. However, about a month prior to this appointment, I noticed something on my back that I had not seen in the past.

It didn't seem like it would be from the radiation, considering this spot was found in the middle of my back. I wasn't even sure how I found it myself. It wasn't easy for me to see.

With my dad's skin cancer in mind, I had some concerns. As always, Dr. N answered all my questions promptly and professionally.

"Maybe I'm more cautious than before my cancer diagnosis, but I noticed a spot on my back that I never noticed before." I lifted the lower half of my gown to show her. "Do you think I should get it checked?"

She leaned into me and looked very carefully at the spot. "Just keep an eye on it. If something unusual shows up anywhere else or this spot increases in size, or changes texture or color, please contact me."

She continued to physically check me all over from the waist up. I was glad she was thorough. One of my biggest fears was the cancer coming back. Dr. N told me that if I did all the treatments recommended by my doctors, and was routinely checked, I should be fine. I continued with the other questions and she patiently answered each one.

"Should I have my white blood cell count checked the next time I get blood work done?"

"You should be fine since you had the white blood cell injections."

"Is it safe for me to get vaccines?" I asked.

"You should get the flu vaccine, but you should wait on the others."

"When should I start the Tamoxifen?"

"You can start at once. I'll prescribe it for you." She typed the order into the computer.

"Now that I'm done, is there a follow-up test that I'll need to see if we got rid of all the cancer? I'm not sure what to tell people as far as my cancer is concerned."

"Another test is not necessary. We say you have 'no evidence of cancer.'"

"Is there anything I can do to reduce the chance of recurrence?"

"You did everything you could to get rid of your cancer. There's no guarantee the cancer will not come back. The Tamoxifen and all the other treatments this year should decrease the chances of it recurring."

I handed her a thank you card. It didn't seem like much since she had done so much for me. I knew it was her job. Then again, not everyone did their job to help me get rid of the cancer. Dr. N always handled my many questions with grace and dignity. And I could not thank her enough for that.

After that appointment, I decided to share a photo of myself holding a sign that said, "No Evidence of Cancer" with many people who had been supporting me throughout the year.

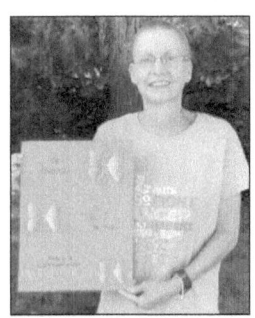

No evidence.
Photo by Mark Ormsby.

Several different people thanked me for letting them know about the positive outcome of my treatment. One person said it was so nice to hear some good news for a change. I hadn't looked at it that way. So glad I sent the message.

As for any side effects of my treatments, my nails never did change from the chemo. Apparently, it doesn't happen to everyone. And if the tissue did shrink at all during radiation, it wasn't obvious to me. Aside from the years of Tamoxifen or some other hormone pills, my tests and treatments were done.

* * *

I was hoping I would gain some much-needed weight during the treatments, especially since I wasn't very sick during chemotherapy. No such luck. However, my weight seemed to be holding steady.

Plus, my mindset had changed, and I was getting used to being slimmer. Finding the right clothes had been a struggle as I was losing weight. Now that I had stopped losing, it was easier to figure out my wardrobe.

I was also feeling more confident in my eating. I was eating bigger portions once in a while and eating more often. I tried protein drinks, too, but they made me too full at mealtimes. Those small changes slightly increased my appetite but still weren't helping me gain weight.

There was something I remembered from my past. When I was in my twenties, I had a live-in nanny job for a big and busy family.

Part of my regimen back then included muffins almost daily. This family bought big packs of muffins, and I was home all day with the babies. Boy, were those muffins ever good! Two years and fifteen pounds later, I realized that muffins can put on some weight!

Because of the pandemic, I couldn't go to the gym to build some muscle back. So, I decided to try the muffin method.

Of course, I was much younger and didn't have diabetes the last time. So, muffins would only be a temporary way to gain weight until I could find a better solution.

It did help a little. After about a month, I was finally back in the triple digits! As good as those muffins tasted, I had to slow down my muffin consumption. Not only was I trying to keep my A1c at a good number, but I also noticed where the added weight was going. If only I could've told the weight where to go.

The real plan was to gain most of my weight back by working out. In other words, once I started working out to burn enough calories, then that would increase my appetite. It would also increase my muscle mass which should, in turn, help me feel stronger.

* * *

Once all my active treatments were done, I was able to do some organizing. Officially, the cleaning started over the summer while I was getting chemo. I asked my two oldest to help by cleaning out many drawers in our basement rec room. There had been items in there for at least ten years.

I also cleaned our den. That was the room I had jokingly referred to as The Abyss. Whenever someone in my family does not know what to do with something, it winds up in the den.

Then I noticed I was having trouble stopping. My organizing continued for some time. Perhaps it was because I wanted 2021 to be as different from 2020 as possible. When I noticed *any* clutter, I had to do something about it.

Out of curiosity, I checked on Google to see if there was any information about cancer treatment and nesting. Sure enough, I stumbled upon something in Debbie Woodbury's blog "Journeying Beyond Breast Cancer" that made perfectly good sense to me.

Who deserves to feather their nest more than the cancer survivor? During the diagnostic and treatment phases, there is no time or energy left for

anything other than dealing with cancer. But little by little, you get stron-
ger and stronger and yearn to reclaim your most intimate places from
the intruder. Nesting re-establishes security, scrubs away sickness, and
reclaims the sanctuary which is your home.

Along with nesting, my recurring dreams started up again. Other cancer survivors had told me that they had vivid dreams while they were receiving chemo. I actually don't remember any dreams during that time.

One dream I had for years always involved seeing myself running through the streets of an unfamiliar city. I would just keep running, street after street, with no idea where I was going. I wasn't even worried. It was like I was so used to feeling that way that I never panicked.

One variant of that dream in late 2020 was that I said out loud to myself, "This can't be a dream. I must really be running because I'm feeling so tired!" Then I woke up.

The other recurring dream I used to have was that I was in a crowd of hundreds and I didn't know anyone there. Again, I wasn't worried. In my dream, it seemed normal for me to be there. It looked like I was joining an event already in progress and I didn't care that I was late.

That time around, my dream also included me showing up to the event and noticing that I was the only one wearing a mask! I was so upset. It was 2020 after all.

* * *

By that time, I had been taking Tamoxifen for about a month. I'm pretty sure that was not the reason for my dreams. However, it did cause occasional stomach issues. For the most part, I was okay taking it. I am the kind of person who seems to have horrible side effects from medicines so I was willing to deal with one effect that was not happening all the time.

Another change for me at that time was my hair. It wasn't coming in any thicker, as I had hoped it would. It was coming in nicely though. I have never had so many compliments on my hair as I did in the last few months of 2020. Well, most of them were compliments, anyway.

That October, when I was on an elevator heading to an appointment, an older woman stepped onto the elevator just before the door closed. I was tired of wearing the chemo caps and started feeling more confident about not covering my head. So, I went for it. I went out in public without covering my head!

However, I was not expecting the conversation that occurred on the elevator that day.

"Are you getting chemo?" the woman asked in a polite tone.

"No. I'm done with chemo."

"Radiation then?"

"Done with that too." I forced a smile behind my mask. Her questions made me feel uncomfortable.

"Oh, okay. Well, good luck with everything."

She looked back at me while she stepped off the elevator. I kept a smile on my face for as long as I could. One thing I know about a person's looks, it's usually more pleasant to see a smile than a frown on their face, even when they are wearing a mask.

I was being polite. I was also trying to look happier and healthier than I was at the time. I'm not sure why that mattered. It just did.

About a week later, I went out again without covering my head. I was standing in line by myself in a store. There were two other customers in front of me, each of us about six feet away from the person in front of them. A woman came in and stepped into line about another six feet behind me.

"Excuse me," said a female voice.

"Yes?" I turned around to see if she was talking to me.

"I love your hair!" she said.

"Thank you so much." I wondered if I should mention the chemo I had earlier that year or if she could already tell.

When it started growing back, more and more I would leave my head uncovered during Zoom sessions and outdoors. Other people who have known me for years complimented me on my hair.

But this was someone I had never met. I was more concerned about possibly embarrassing her if she didn't know I had cancer. Then I decided to take a chance.

"Actually...I had chemo over the summer. It's still growing back."

"Well, it looks great! I love the way it looks in the back with your neckline. You can get away with keeping your hair very short. It's a good look on you."

That was one of the sincerest compliments I ever had in my life. And for someone to compliment me on my hair was even better. I have never liked my hair. My sister went through chemo years before me. When I first found out I would need chemo, and would definitely be losing my hair, I told her. Her reply was interesting.

"We're Dutcher women. We don't have thick and gorgeous hair, so losing it isn't very traumatic anyway."

I'm not sure I really agreed with her. In hindsight, it wasn't so bad after all. And it was definitely easier to take care of with it shorter.

- 8 -

Shared Moments

It was early November 2020. Donna invited Jill and me to lunch again. This time, she asked if we could go closer to her home. I didn't know that she had been traveling from another state for her treatments. She used to live much closer to where we were getting radiation, so she had already established a team of doctors in that area.

Jill couldn't make that lunch but, especially considering Donna was having a hard time with her chemo treatments, I didn't mind heading down to her area. Once she was up to eating again, we met for lunch. It was cold outside. Unfortunately, we couldn't eat inside because the pandemic was still going strong.

Despite the cold, we enjoyed our lunch together, then warmed up by going somewhere else for hot chocolate. It was a nice way to spend the afternoon.

That day Donna explained that she had been getting chemo every Monday for seven weeks, which altered her radiation schedule on Mondays, and that was why we only saw her then. Aside from looking a little thinner, she still looked amazing considering what she had been through.

* * *

I had my annual eye exam just before Thanksgiving. Unlike previous years, that time I was wearing a mask. The place I went to was inside a mall. Since the pandemic hit locally, I had not entered any mall in the seven months leading up to this appointment. While I was there, I told my optometrist about my cancer. We discovered that we had the same medical oncologist. What a small world!

* * *

Being that my relatives all live far away from me and my family, we had some Zoom sessions with them during the later 2020 holidays. Considering many people went without haircuts during the pandemic, and I had lost my hair, that topic came up a couple of times in our online gatherings. During our Thanksgiving Zoom, one of my brothers commented on my hair.

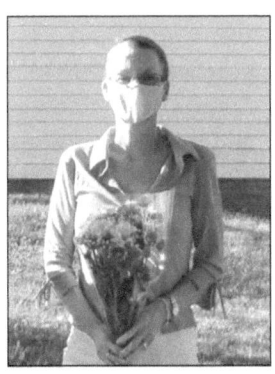

Thankful for life.
Photo by Erin Ormsby

"Wendy, I love that you're keeping your hair short!" he said with a smile.

"I love that you *think* I'm keeping my hair short. I haven't cut it yet." I smiled back at him.

Thanksgiving 2020 was not the same as other years, but my family was still able to enjoy our traditional Thanksgiving dinner together at home. Our oldest child, who had been going by a different name up until then, sprang some news on us over the holiday.

As my husband and I were preparing our Thanksgiving meal, out of the blue our child said to call them Ezra and use the pronouns they/them from now on. It was stressful at first. I was still recovering from treatments, and it was a lot to think about. But it was important to our child. That's all that really mattered. We eventually acclimated.

❋ ❋ ❋

Every year I write my family's holiday letter that sums up our year and send it to many people we've met over the years. Some years I wrote a poem. Other years I designed a collage and let the photos speak for themselves.

The year 2020 was especially difficult. At first, I wasn't sure how much to say about my health. After all, it was a *holiday* letter. Then I realized my health is what my year was about more than anything. There was no way to ignore "the elephant in the room."

That one turned out to be the easiest holiday letter I have ever put together. Since our family couldn't do nearly as much as we usually did because of my treatments and COVID, there weren't many photos. The same concept applied to the narrative. I was able to write a few things about each person and include a few photos with the comments.

The best idea I could come up with for myself was to be informative but not elaborate too much about my cancer. I didn't mention that I was writing this book. However, I did say something about other side projects that helped me get through my treatments. I kept it short and sweet.

* * *

I was hoping to get my COVID vaccine soon after the 2020 holidays. While I was waiting to qualify for the vaccine, something tragic happened to my friend Shobha and her husband Bill. They were both diagnosed with COVID, and Bill ended up in the hospital after a few days.

Shobha had a mild case of it. Unfortunately, Bill did not. The two weeks or so he spent in the hospital confirmed something about my family's church. I have never seen so much support and love poured out for two people as I did for Bill and Shobha.

They were cofounders of our church, which started in 1982. It was just them and a pastor and his wife. Our church has grown so much since then.

No matter who you were, Bill and Shobha always showed you their unconditional love and support. They also took the time to listen to each person no matter what they wanted to talk about. Bill and Shobha have touched so many lives over the years.

When Shobha started telling others about Bill going to the hospital with COVID, word spread quickly. While he was hospitalized, friends and loved ones dropped care packages off at their home. Shobha was so appreciative of everything.

On March 5, 2021, the one-year anniversary of the first reported COVID cases in our immediate area, Bill passed away. He was the first friend I lost to the pandemic. Shobha was at his side, holding his hand, and that was all he asked for in the end.

- 9 -

Bittersweet

THERE HAD ALREADY BEEN CONSTANT REMINDERS OF THE PAN-demic everywhere I went. It was especially noticeable at my many medical appointments. The fear of catching COVID was always lingering in the back of my mind. Losing a friend to it encouraged me to look further into getting vaccinated.

I started looking more thoroughly for places to schedule my vaccination. Of course, what held me back was how slowly the phases progressed. We live in a very populated area. The vaccine supply was not a match for the demand.

Johns Hopkins was offering vaccines to those who qualified. I checked online to see if I qualified yet. I was discouraged immediately because they said, along with being a patient of theirs, you must qualify for the current phase. I was too young for that phase.

And, if that wasn't challenging enough, they were choosing patients through a "randomized computer lottery." I've never had much luck playing the lottery. Then, on March 18, 2021,

I received a MyChart message from Johns Hopkins. I couldn't believe what was happening. It really did feel like I won the lottery.

> We want to offer you the chance to schedule an appointment for the COVID-19 vaccine. Please log in to your Johns Hopkins Medicine MyChart account to schedule your appointment. This scheduling ticket is good for the next 10 days.
>
> If you do not schedule your appointment within this time frame, you will automatically be placed back into the randomized computer lottery, and you will need to receive a new scheduling ticket when more vaccine supply is available.

I have never been so nervous about scheduling an appointment in my life! If I made even one mistake, I was afraid I would lose my appointment and be put back into the system. What a crazy feeling. Thankfully, I was able to get my first vaccine five days later. Wow!

* * *

Two days after my first vaccine, I had another follow-up with my surgeon. It had been about thirteen months since my lumpectomy surgery. Dr. S checked me over thoroughly.

"You seem perfectly healthy to me," she confirmed.

"That's great," I replied.

"You don't have to come back for another year. You can also make your appointment with the nurse practitioner."

"Okay."

Hearing this news was bittersweet. On one hand, I was

relieved she didn't find anything new. On the other hand, an overwhelming feeling of sadness came over me later that day. What Dr. S said meant that I most likely wouldn't be seeing her for at least two more years.

As tired as I was of medical appointments by then, I enjoyed being her patient. She took very good care of me. Plus, she was the second out of three from my cancer team whom I wouldn't see again for at least another year.

* * *

A few weeks later, I was given my second COVID vaccine. I had chills during the first two nights and a fever the first two days following my vaccine. I knew that meant it was working. My body was fighting it, and my immune system was strong!

To stay healthy and strong, I would go for walks by myself as a form of meditation. It was much calmer when I walked alone because I didn't have a big distraction from my dogs.

Every day it was not raining, I went on a walk through our neighborhood. Since it was spring, I would stop and notice the flowers and trees that were in bloom. I even took some photos of our scenic neighborhood. I was cancer-free. At least, as cancer-free as I could be. And I was fully vaccinated and did not have COVID-19.

I learned a lot about my health.

I also learned a lot about myself. It's okay to disagree with how you are treated as a patient at times. A doctor is someone you should be able to count on to help heal you and get you through some difficult times with your health. If that doesn't happen, then be your own advocate. Don't be afraid to ask questions, no matter how trivial they may seem. Most importantly, I now realize that I am willing and able to go to great lengths to be healthy again. What a difference between what I knew then and what I know now.

Sources

"My Breast Cancer Treatment, The Oncotype DX Test: Essential Genomic Information for Improving Your Treatment Decision for Early-Stage Invasive Breast Cancer," Genomic Health, Inc., a wholly owned subsidiary of Exact Sciences Corporation, 2020 (accessed 24 April 2020).

www.mybreastcancertreatment.org/en-US/Learn AboutOncotypeDX/WhatIsOncotypeDXForBreastCancer

"State Guidance on Elective Surgeries, Maryland," Ambulatory Surgery Center Association and ASCA Foundation, April 20, 2020 (accessed 12 July 2020).

https://www.ascassociation.org/asca/resourcecenter/ latestnewsresourcecenter/covid-19/covid-19-state

Debbie Woodbury, "Cancer and the Nesting Instinct," Journeying Beyond Breast Cancer (blog), May 24, 2016 (accessed 15 December 2020).

https://journeyingbeyondbreastcancer.com/2016/05/24/ cancer-and-the-nesting-instinct/

About the Author

Wendy Ormsby resides in Maryland with her husband, three young adult children, and their two dogs. She is a teaching assistant in a special education program and the owner of Ormsby Graphics design company.

www.ingramcontent.com/pod-product-compliance
Lightning Source LLC
Chambersburg PA
CBHW020412130626
46549CB00006B/2526